Delay Don't Deprive

Intermittent Fasting: Getting Leaner Without Hunger

Table of Contents

Introduction

When you hear your stomach grumble, you probably want to eat whatever food that is closest to you. Knowing how horrible you feel when you are hungry, you might think you could never fast! If it's not something you regularly do for health or religion, why start now?

Well, that's the great thing about intermittent fasting. It is one of the easiest ways to get healthy and lean. So, what is intermittent fasting? Intermittent fasting is the intentional skipping of one or multiple meals for the amazing benefits that come with it. There are multiple methods of intermittent fasting and the more you do it, the less hunger you will feel during fasting! Intermittent fasting can help you with your weight loss, your heart health, your energy levels, and even help to stabilize your insulin. We'll go over all of this in depth in this book.

If you've tried to do intermittent fasting before, a simple Google search probably came up with a bunch of contradicting and hard to understand articles. You shouldn't need a doctorate degree to understand why you should try intermittent fasting! That's why this book is created. This book aims to break down the mind boggling intermittent fasting information into easy to understand parts that go through every essential aspect of fasting. Not only the pros and cons of intermittent fasting are shared, you will also learn about the history of why fasting started, the science behind fasting, why you should fast for your health, and how you can start intermittent fasting using the right personalized method amongst the different fasting methods.

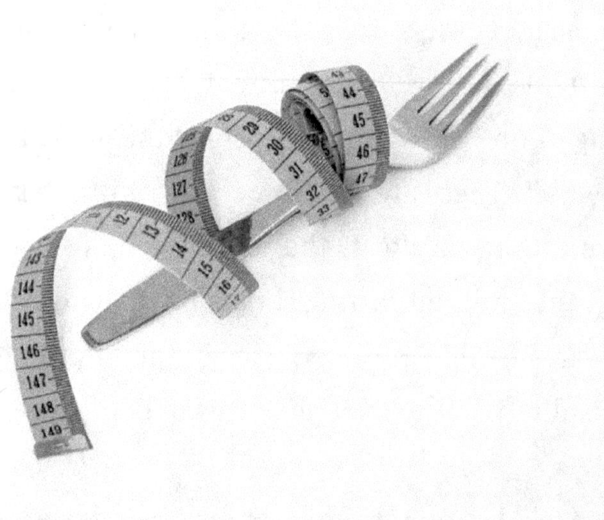

No longer do you have to be lost when searching for how to start intermittent fasting online. This book will become your number one resource to convince you, your family, and your friends that intermittent fasting is easy and healthy. All your questions will be answered and fasting steps will be setup for you in an easy way so you can get started immediately. Keep reading on to learn how intermittent fasting can help you get the lean and healthy body you have ever wanted.

Part One

Fasting: Understanding the Basics

Chapter 1: What Causes Obesity?

With the development of more diets than ever and countless low-fat products on the grocery store shelves, you would think that people in urban civilizations are the healthiest they have ever been. In reality, the overall human race is now the unhealthiest ever been. Obesity is on the rise and we now have higher rates of heart disease, high blood pressure, and obesity related deaths. In fact, one third of the American population is obese! One in every three people are considered obese. And over half of the population is overweight. The numbers are staggering and yet people are not losing the weight they need to, so they can live a happy and healthy life. Why is this?

Obesity comes with a long range of problems. From sleep apnea to death, obesity messes with our health. Despite us knowing that being obese can be just as bad as smoking a pack of cigarettes a day, society is not making substantial change. Key is that most people find it near impossible to change their "comfortable" lifestyle which has been so deeply ingrained into them since birth with their family eating culture and habits.

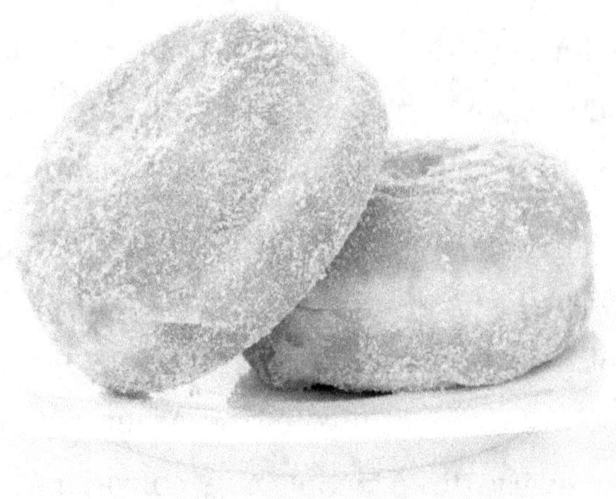

Eating more calories than you expend generally causes obesity. Throughout the day and night, your body burns calories. Calories are like the gas human body needs to run on. We need a certain amount of calories to keep our bodies functioning at their optimal level throughout the day. We burn calories all day while walking around, digesting food, breathing, and even sleeping! Every function of our body requires calories. You can easily calculate your daily caloric need by adding your basal metabolic rate, the amount of food you eat, and the thermal effect of food (this is the calories you burn while digesting your food). Any physical activity you do beyond your normal day, causes you to burn, or expend, more calories. That is why if you want to lose weight you need to expend more calories and work out so that you create a calorie deficit. But if you eat more calories than you expend, you will gain fats while breathing and even sleeping! Over the years with such cycles of calorie surplus, you will be gradually gaining fat while losing muscle, which leads to obesity. If you are consuming 1,300 calories more than you need, you will be gaining an extra pound every 3 days. See how easy it is to put on extra weight without realizing it?

To stop gaining weight and start losing weight, a calorie deficit has to be created. Exercises like weight lifting and high intensity interval training are workouts most effective in creating the largest calorie deficit.

Typically, most people gain weight due to poor diets and poor food choices. They often find themselves eating processed food high in trans-fat and sugar. Certain medical conditions like lack of thyroid function, polycystic ovarian syndrome, and some medications may cause extra weight too. Genetics may also be a factor for weight gain. If your family all has insatiable appetites, you may have been blessed with it too! But, while these conditions can lead to weight gain, they do not lead to obesity.

It is still possible to lose weight with these conditions and with poor genetics.

The extra calories are stored in the form of fat in our body as a survival mechanism biologically. In other words, on days when we eat more than needed, our body will store the excess energy as fat thinking that there is a chance of having days without food (think of the caveman hunting era).

So how do our body store fat exactly? Well, fat cells are cells that contain extra calories to use subsequently. These fat stores are called adipose tissue. Fat is a nutrient needed for our body function. Besides providing energy for our daily functions, it also provides energy for the biochemical actions within the body. If we do not have fat, our body organs would be subjected to degradation. However, we do not need huge excess amount of fat too. Hence, just like stone age cavemen hunt food to survive, we exercise to build healthy muscles and use up these fat storage cells. This will have our fat to get exhaled during work-out while oxygen is inhaled.

So that's about it for the technical part of how our body handles fat. Moving on, more about history of fasting and various types of fasting practiced today will be shared.

Chapter 2: History of Fasting

Fasting is something that has been practiced by different cultures and religions. Fasting is conversely a survival instinct that has been with us since the beginning of time. Humans and animals alike can be found fasting during periods of stress, illness, or for survival. Fasting occurs when food and/or drink is for a period of time. It is a natural instinct that we practice when our bodies crave rest or when we want to conserve energy for a later time. But besides fasting for survival, where did fasting come from?

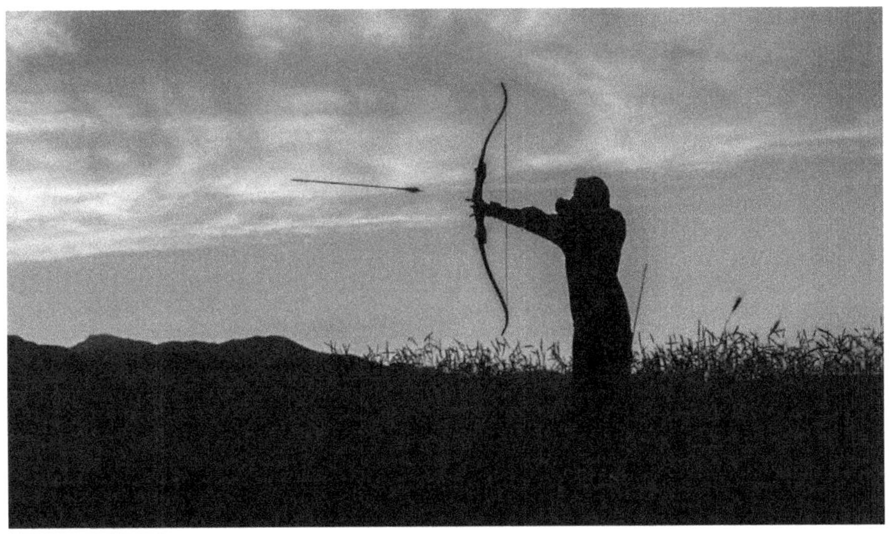

Fasting for spiritual purposes dates back thousands of

years. While many religions practice fasting, the reasons behind it are about the same. Most fast for spiritual strength. When their mind is turned away from food and drink, they can focus more heavily on things they need to atone for or recognize. Fasting was used before war and big events. People also believed that fasting could be used for healing of the body.

Christians devote their fasting towards Christ. Jesus Christ fasted for 40 days and nights and created a fasting regimen for others to follow for religious strength. Judaism has Yom Kippur fasting where they fast for one whole day to atone for your sins of the previous year. Muslims fast for the whole month of Ramadan where they do not eat from sun up to sun down. Native American tribes would fast to avoid potential natural disasters. There are also other fasts in many religions not mentioned.

As such, fasting isn't an abnormal or un-natural behavior. It has been around and shown to be beneficial for the body and mind as practiced by various religions and cultures.

Chapter 3: Why You Should Fast

You do not need to fast for your survival, and you may or may not fast for your religion. So, if it is not required due to such religious or survival reasons, why would you want to fast? While fasting has often been closely tied to religion, it has become far more popular in recent years. You may have heard people talking about different forms of fasting and how it relates to their diet. You may even have a friend who claims fasting is the greatest new thing! Before you scoff and call these friends crazy, there are surprisingly many beneficial health reasons for you to fast. There is a reason why many people called fasting the physician within your body! Fasting brings about balance to your body and promotes healing from within. What are these benefits and how can you get them?

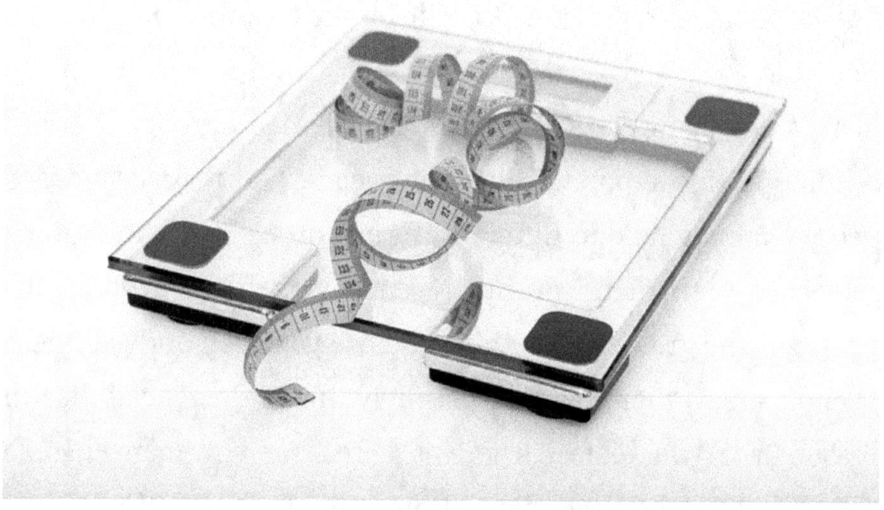

The first benefit that may be obvious is that fasting helps with weight loss. It should come as no surprise that fasting helps you to eat fewer calories. When you are skipping meals or skipping days of eating, you are going to be eating fewer calories throughout the day. As long as you don't binge eat when you stop fasting, you'll start to see weight loss. This is because you are expending more calories than you are eating throughout the day. Research has shown that individuals who practiced intermittent fasting while trying to lose weight actually lost up to 10% of their body weight and lost fat in their stomachs. Losing weight from intermittent fasting can help halt your progress of weight related diseases like type 2 diabetes, heart disease, and cancer. If you are looking to lose weight, intermittent fasting is a great method to cut out calories without having to try to find a healthy meal replacement.

Improve Heart Health

Another reason you should try intermittent fasting is that it can help to maintain healthy heart! Obesity is one of the top causes for heart disease and heart attacks. When individuals are overweight, their hearts have to pump much harder to keep their body working. Heart is a muscle that also can get tired! When one is overweight, there will be additional stress on the heart.

Intermittent fasting helps to reverse obesity and thus helps the heart pump blood better; reduce the risk of cardiac arrhythmia, heart disease and heart attack. As an easy positive health indicator is that after a period of fasting practice (at least 6 months), one can usually see blood pressure decrease. This is especially important if you find that individuals in your family have had heart attacks or who have gone into cardiac arrest. Intermittent fasting is negatively correlated with your morbidity risk. This means that when you fast, you have a lower chance of dying.

When you wake up the day after Halloween after eating half of the candy you bought to hand out for trick or treaters, how do you feel? Most often, you feel sick in your stomach, sluggish, and just gross! You may have even gone as far as saying you need to detox or do a cleanse. These cleanses and detox diets on the market today might not be the best solutions for everyone. On the other hand, intermittent fasting can easily be used as a detox method. If you are feeling sluggish and dull, look to intermittent fasting to fix these things. Imagine you are pressing a reset button on your body! Every day our bodies are filled with chemicals, toxins, and hard to digest food. Our body is constantly trying to digest the food we put in our body that it cannot focus on cleansing and detoxing itself. That is why we need to do intermittent fasting. Intermittent fasting allows our bodies to focus more on detoxing. It can forget about the energy it needs to devote to your metabolism for digestion and use that energy elsewhere. Many people report after intermittent fasting to feeling relaxed and rejuvenated. They feel their body has taken on a whole new experience and they feel much better. After days, weeks, or months of not detoxing, our bodies become slow. They have to work that much harder to get simple things done.

Reduce Food Attachment

What do most of us think about all day? Food! We are a slave to our metabolisms. While we need food to survive, we have all changed to survive solely for food. Food is a big part of what we do throughout the day. We plan every meal; we constantly think about that next snack, we literally do everything for our next meal. This should not be how it is! Instead of choosing food to help us become healthy, we constantly look for the next best food. We crave those ice cream sundaes at fast food restaurants and when something like a cronut or rainbow bagel hits the market, thousands of people flood those stores for a chance to eat the newest food available. This is exhausting on our bodies and minds! If we want to cut the ball and chain attached to our ankle, we must do so by not letting food control us. We want freedom from food! Intermittent fasting can provide that as a solution for us. When you fast, you realize that you can amazingly survive without food for a period of time. It is not going to kill you when you have a meal skipped. In fact, it allows you the freedom from food that you seek! When you realize that you do not need the food right when you think about it, you stop being a slave to your metabolism. The more you practice intermittent fasting, the more you recognize that your life should not be dependent on your next meal. You can focus your energy on more important things.

Anti-aging

It may seem counterintuitive that eating less provides more energy. However, this is true! When we eat, our body gets an increase in insulin and our body gathers energy up to digest the food. Do you ever feel tired after eating? You think you should have more energy after lunch but sometimes you feel like you need a nap! That's because your insulin levels are on a rollercoaster. A little more about this will be shared below but for now imagine your body is filled with sugar. You then hit the inevitable sugar crash. This happens when you eat. When you put carbohydrates into your body, your brain takes them and uses them. The problem with carbs is that they burn out quickly. They are not a stable energy force. This cycle happens every time you eat. You end up becoming hungrier, more frustrated, and more tired every time. So how does intermittent fasting change this? Intermittent fasting changes the way you get your energy. Because you are not eating as often, your body starts burning fat instead of carbohydrates. While this is also beneficial for weight loss, it improves your brain functions as well. You see, your brain loves carbohydrates, but they aren't all that good for it. Instead, fat is more stable and allows your brain to function better. Intermittent fasting allows your brain to use fat instead of carbs as energy fuel. What you get is a smoother and more even performance. Instead of going up and down in your energy, it stays stable. This provides more energy and you'll feel rejuvenated and refreshed after you eat instead of immediately crashing. This can also help in aging backwards. Not only are you going to feel younger with more energy, but also having this energy allows your brain to begin a process called autophagy. This is where your old cells can repair themselves into healthy new cells. This process of switching metabolism into utilizing ketones from glucose will then help anti-aging.

Stabilize Insulin

Evidently, insulin stabilization is another great benefit of intermittent fasting. Insulin by itself is not inherently bad. Insulin is needed for body function and survival. However, when insulin rises, fat is stored in our cells and cannot be utilized as energy. Every time food is consumed, insulin level will be increased. While exercise is always the most beneficial way to decrease or stabilize insulin levels, intermittent fasting can help even more. When our insulin levels are constantly rising and falling when we eat, we are left feeling exhausted. Not only tiredness plagues us, such insulin roller coaster rides also cause us to be fat! When you take food away during fasting, your insulin levels decrease. This is good because it leads to lower blood sugar levels, which decrease your risk for diseases like type 2 diabetes. You'll also increase your fat burning abilities and have more energy from fewer spikes in your insulin.

As illustrated, fasting is not only a religious practice. Fasting can miraculously help to achieve your health goals! There are so many benefits to fasting and creating a healthy diet. You can reduce your risk of many diseases and increase your longevity.

Chapter 4: My First Fasting Experience

Even though there are tons of benefits to fasting, your first time doing it may not be the most pleasant experience. Let me share what I have gone through when I tried intermittent fasting for the first time. There are some positive and negative things that happen as you embark this unique intermittent fasting journey and integrate as part of your lifestyle.

I'm not going to lie, those first few days when I started intermittent fasting were really challenging on my mind! My brain was probably constantly sending signals that it "needs" food. Conversely, it does not actually need food but it sure felt like it did. Everyone else's food around me was evidently noticed unfortunately. Coworker is eating shrimp? I may hate shrimp but all of a sudden that smelled delicious. Literally everything I did had me thinking of food! It was a rough few days for my mind. Thus, if you know about this ahead of time, you can prepare better for it and be ready when the time comes.

It should also come as no surprise that your stomach is going to give you grief. You are about to sound like a whale is mating in your stomach. It is going to grumble at arena event volume.

This will of course make you feel like you are starving! Do not worry, this is also temporary. I like to call the first few days of intermittent fasting the adjustment period. Your body goes a little crazy! Be prepared to have a super loud stomach. That's not all the physical symptoms you'll experience. You are also going to be tired, more irritable, and you'll probably even feel like you are betraying your body. Do not, I repeat, do not give up! This is completely and totally temporary.

If you want a baseline before you start intermittent fasting, weigh yourself, figure out your body percentage, and then get some blood tests done. When you get blood work done, you can see your cholesterol levels and different hormones in your body. It is not a must, but it is nice to see what your body weight improved on besides energy and weight loss.

Once your body adjusts and understands that you are not in fact trying to kill it, some crazy things happen! The biggest thing I did not expect with intermittent fasting is the amount of energy and focus I have. I am not only more energized, I feel like my thinking is clearer. When I work throughout the day I do not have to think nearly as hard and I have become a lot more productive. This makes my work day easier and I get more things done! Because I am more productive throughout my day, I also become a lot more relaxed and patient. When a coworker comes to me with a problem, I'm not worried about the time it is taking because I know my work is still going to get done. This was an amazing mental benefit from starting my intermittent fasting. It was also incredible to see how much stress was reduced. My mind reacts better to situations and feels more composed in challenging situations.

Physically, I could tell a lot of difference from my body after I started to do intermittent fasting. Of course, there was weight loss but I did not expect the fat loss and muscle gain that happened. I have worked for years to get my visceral fat from my stomach to go away. I've tried every diet and every exercise on the market. I finally accepted that I was just doomed to have a stomach pouch the rest of my life. I almost gave up trying to get rid of it. After a few weeks of intermittent fasting, I could see my stomach shrinking! I didn't even want to get my hopes up in case it was a fluke! But sure enough, when I went to my doctor, my body fat percentage had gone down. Even though I had not changed my exercise routine, my body fat went down, and I started to finally lose that stomach pouch. The only thing I did differently was added in intermittent fasting!

I chose to get my blood work done before I started intermittent fasting because my family has always had the risk of high cholesterol. I figured if intermittent fasting could help me lower my cholesterol, then why not? I waited three months between getting my blood work done the first time and the second time. The second time I'd been doing intermittent fasting for two months. I was shocked when I saw that my cholesterol had lowered. My parents take medication to keep their cholesterol lowered and I immediately called them up and told them my results! They were shocked and asked me to help them start intermittent fasting for them as well. My triglycerides had also lowered which is never a bad thing!

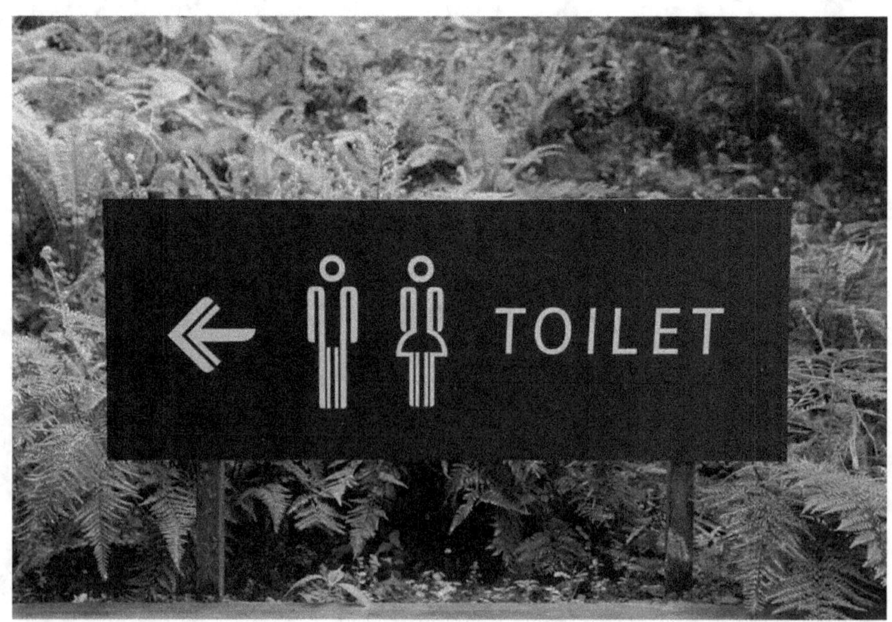

Now, I'm going to get a little personal with you here. One thing I did not expect from intermittent fasting was what it did to my digestion track. You will find that you will be going to the bathroom regularly. And what I mean by that is, you will find yourself making a trip to the bathroom at the same time every day. This is obviously a benefit for people who struggle with constipation. Intermittent fasting has made it so I never have to take constipation medicine or added fiber again. When I take a trip to the bathroom, it's quick, easy, and dependable. I don't want to talk about it too much, just know that you are about to become a daily regular to your bathroom seat!

The thing I was most worried about when starting intermittent fasting was my exercise routine. I've worked out on an empty stomach before and I have always felt faint and light headed. When I worked out at the beginning of intermittent fasting, I felt like my workout surely suffered. I felt weak and sluggish and had a hard time getting through it. For me now, I work out best in my fasted state. It depends on what intermittent fasting routine you use for sure. I like to exercise in the mornings and I fast most mornings. Sometimes my exercise is still hard. I still have days I feel more sluggish or tired. On these days sometimes, I will work out after I've eaten. You have to find what works best for you and fits your lifestyle. Not everyone can work out while fasting but not everyone can work out after eating a large meal either. It's really a personal choice and you have to feel it out for yourself. I don't think my workout regime has suffered at all though now. It's just different.

My key advice here is that when you first start intermittent fasting, you are going to experience harmless side effects. The important part of this is to keep your mind occupied and not to give up. Whenever you feel like quitting, think of why you started it. Do not think that intermittent fasting is only battling hunger. It should not be! Be optimistic and intermittent fasting will simply get better and easier over time. Make sure that when you try intermittent fasting, you give it at least a month trial before deciding if it's not for you.

Chapter 5: Who Should Avoid Fasting?

Fasting may be beneficial for most people. Unfortunately, it may not be a one size fits all type of program. While it boasts many different health benefits, there are some people who may not be suited for fasting. Fasting can harm some individuals so always check to make sure you do not have any underlying medical conditions before fasting.

Medical Conditions

Individuals who are not healthy in a mental or physical aspect should not try fasting. If you find that you have a lot of mental stressors in your life, put fasting on the back burner. This does not mean you couldn't plan to engage intermittent fasting later on, but until your mind is ready, it's best to skip fasting. If in doubt, always check out with your doctor for clearance.

Highly Intensive Workouts

If you have any risk of being frail or malnourished, fasting won't be beneficial for you. This also goes to say that if you are exercising intensively every day, fasting might not be that suitable for you. You may still proceed but special efforts have to be made to plan your meals macronutrients and micronutrients intake to ensure you are sufficiently nourished and energy well replenished.

Pregnancy and Breastfeeding

While there is conflicting information out there, pregnant and breastfeeding women should try to avoid regular fasting. While fasting every once in a while will not hurt, consistent fasting, like with intermittent fasting, can affect your nutrients intake for your baby or lower your milk supply. Once you have delivered and stopped breastfeeding, you can benefit better from intermittent fasting.

Diabetics

Diabetics should also be wary of fasting. While people with type two diabetes may benefit from fasting, it can be very dangerous for a type one diabetic. If your diet is currently insulin controlled, do not start fasting unless you have discussed with your medical provider. Fasting can lead to weight loss and stabilization of insulin, which could help type two diabetics but you need to be aware of how it could affect your insulin in a controlled diet. It is critical to consult professional medical advice before proceeding.

High Cortisol

If you are stressed or dealing with high levels of cortisol in your body, you should not fast. Whether you are monitoring your cortisol levels professionally or just noticing the extra stomach fat combined with your high stress levels, its best to clear yourself from the condition before fasting. Fasting raises your cortisol levels. While this is fine in people with normal cortisol levels, if you are already high on cortisol this can lead to more weight gain and added stress.

Children

Also, children should not fast. Intermittent fasting is great for adults but children need proper nutrition intake throughout the day to help their growing bodies.

Other Medical Conditions

Other disorders like kidney disease; anemia, frequent fainting, and liver disease are all other important reasons to avoid fasting. Check with your doctor if you have one of these diseases.

And finally, if you have any history of disordered eating, fasting should be avoided completely. Because of the mental stress fasting can cause, it's recommended that anyone who previously has had an eating disorder should abstain from fasting.

While the majority people can safely fast, always take notice of your medical conditions and ask your doctor if fasting is best for you.

Chapter 6: Fasting Drawbacks

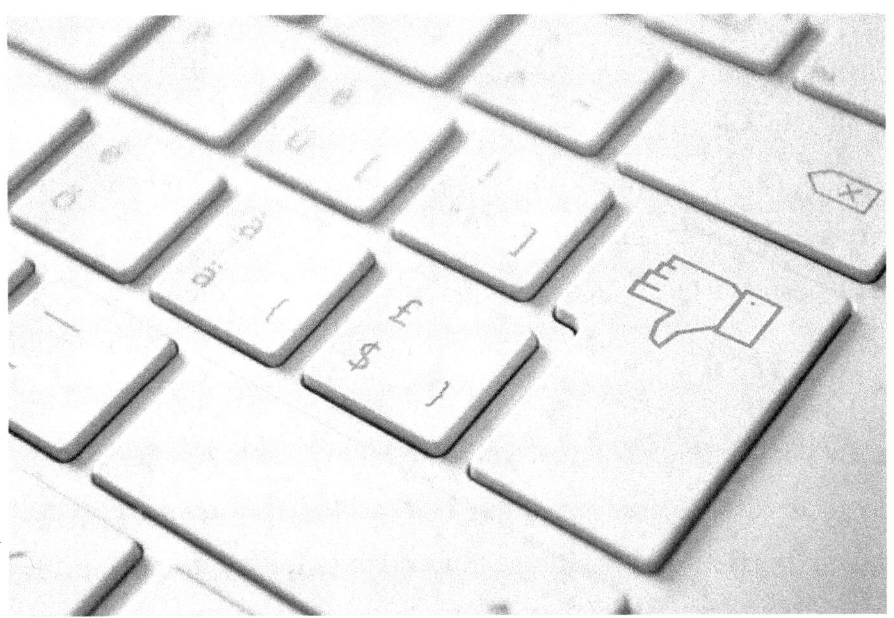

As with any new fitness regimen or diet, intermittent fasting is not always perfect. Some benefits were shared in previous chapters and more will be mentioned subsequently as well. However, fasting definitely comes with some drawbacks that beginners need to be aware of.

Before going into the research studies that have found great success with intermittent fasting, it is worth noting that there are limited long-term studies about the benefits of fasting for extended period of time. Due to this lack of long-term research, some may not find it convincing enough to try out fasting.

Fasting also comes with a slew of other drawbacks. While you will lose weight and gain some health benefits, you may go through a hard transition period. Many people find that they are not used to fasting. If you have never fasted before, the experience is going to be challenging for the first few times. The transition period causes endless thoughts of every food you can dream of. You're going to want to devour everything in sight but then you'll remember that you can't! This transition period also leads to intense cravings. Your body will try to signal you that it needs nutrients by sending you cravings for high fat and high sugar items like chocolate cake. This is because your brain will be notified from its neurotransmitters that it is lacking certain energy that comes from your calories. Thus, your brain will try to flood your synapses with chemicals that will make you want the highest calorie thing available to quickly give your brain energy. However, your brain doesn't actually need these calories. It is just signaling you because that's what it is used to. You will find that when the first few rough patch days are passed, you won't have those intense cravings anymore.

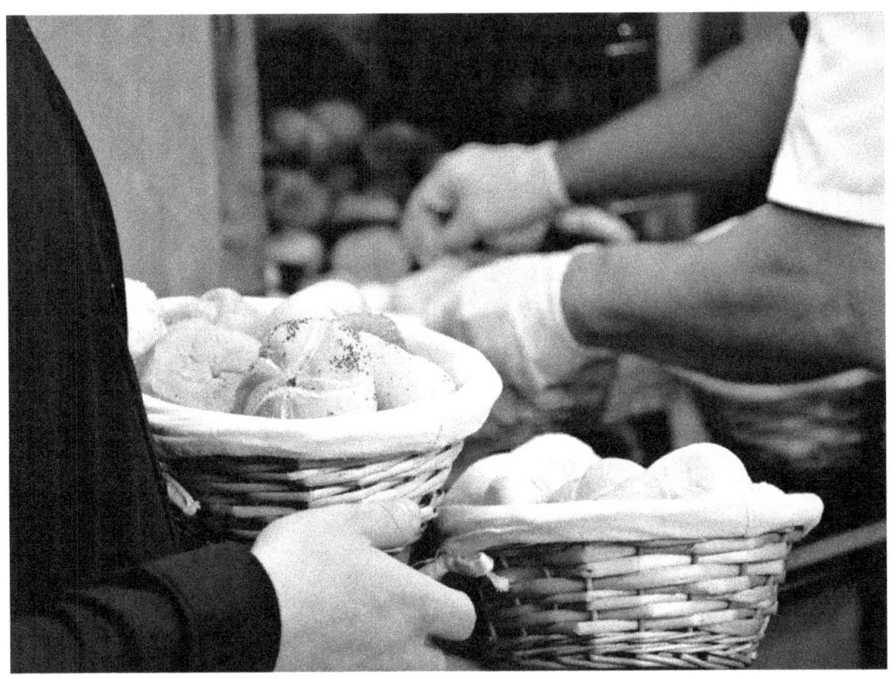

The beginning of your fasting journey can also lead to your body feeling sluggish and lagging. You may feel a loss of energy and light headed. Your body is so used to being fed every few hours that these signs and symptoms will happen because your insulin is down. But this is actually a good thing. Once your insulin is leveled out you'll find that you will get more energy back than you started with.

Once you've been fasting for a while, your body gets used to this. If you skip breakfast every morning while fasting but then decide to have breakfast one day, you are going to suffer some consequences. Your insulin will spike, your blood sugar will rise, and you may feel like you have a brick in your stomach. After eating, you are going to hit an insulin crash and vow to not eat breakfast again. This can be a downside for some people if they like to switch up their routine often. Intermittent fasting does the best if you are consistent in your eating timings.

Another unpleasant effect of intermittent fasting is the associated increased stress. Fasting can be stressful on your body and on your mind! You may be worried about when you get to eat next and not eating can cause you to be stressed over small things. When you are tired or hungry, you are often quicker to snap at things because your brain is not functioning at its highest capacity. While your stress will most likely go down as you continue to fast, adding another potential stressor to your life is something you should consider and plan carefully.

Chapter 7: What Science Says

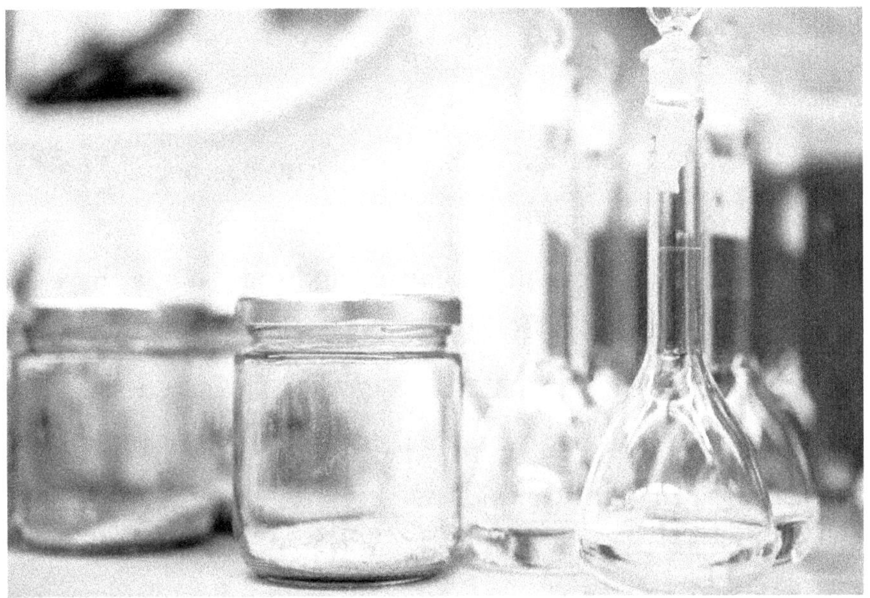

While every diet and fitness addition into your life comes with upsides and downsides, intermittent fasting has more pros than cons. If you approach intermittent fasting with an open mind, you'll find that it can help you reach your weight loss goals. In the next part more will be shared about the science behind intermittent fasting and what you can do about your hunger while fasting.

There is plenty of information and research that backs up intermittent fasting. As fasting is not a new thing, extensive research can be found on this topic. Intermittent fasting may soon become a fad, but thankfully it is a fad that is based in science. While much of the research on fasting has been done on animals, the science is still promising.

Fasting is not a new phenomenon. Fasting has been shown in the past to help the body to reset and clear the mind. Interestingly, the science goes far beyond that. While there are several different theories as to why intermittent fasting works, one fascinating theory that has been well-researched is that intermittent fasting puts your body's cells under a mild stress. When these cells are stressed they keep adapting and can fight off disease better. Stress is something that often carries a negative connotation. On the contrary, stress is not inherently a bad thing. When you put your body under stress, positive results can occur. Think of when you exercise hard. You are exhausted and tired but once your muscles recover, they are stronger. Research has shown that your body's cells respond to intermittent fasting very similar to exercise.

The reason you will lose weight while intermittent fasting can be attributed to a few different causes. For one, it will be much easier to eat fewer calories in the limited eating window. If you are eating on alternate days, during a window period, or skipping certain meals, you will tend to be consuming fewer calories than when you were eating multiple meals throughout the day. Another reason you may lose weight while fasting is because when you stop eating for an extended period of time, your body goes into its adipose tissue fat cells for energy. Ketones are released into the bloodstream that carries fat and you end up losing your body fat through your urine. Research also shows that short term fasting actually increases your metabolism speed. Your metabolism is what digests your food. When it works faster, it burns more calories leading to more weight lost. While many other diets may limit your calorie intake, intermittent fasting does both things. You increase your calories you expend (by boosting your metabolism) and you also decrease the calories you eat. This creates a large calorie deficit. If you exercise on top of intermittent fasting, your calorie deficit becomes larger and you will lose even more weight.

Intermittent fasting did not become a craze just because of weight loss. Intermittent fasting is popular among many already fit individuals because of the other benefits it comes with. One of these benefits is reducing the chance of insulin resistance. Type two diabetes is on the rise. Research says that intermittent fasting actually leads to a drop in blood sugar levels. Fasting insulin was seen to drop as much as 20-30% and fasting blood sugar dropped by 3-6%. When you have lower insulin and blood sugar levels, you are at a lower risk for developing insulin resistance, which leads to type two diabetes.

If you are looking for anti-aging benefits, intermittent fasting may be the diet for you too. Our bodies go through a process called oxidative stress. Oxidative stress leads to aging and many of the chronic diseases that we see on the rise today. Harmful free radicals react with our body's proteins and DNA and damage them which leads to these diseases and aging. However, studies have shown that intermittent fasting actually increases our body's ability to attack these harmful free radicals. This can help us to combat the effects of aging.

Fasting is also good for heart. It's no surprise that cardiovascular disease is currently the number one killer in many countries. Intermittent fasting can help stabilize brain's hormones and brings about better heart health. Fasting can reduce risk of heart problems with risk factors such as LDL cholesterol, blood triglycerides, blood sugar levels, and inflammation levels lowered. If you have high cholesterol or are on medication for cholesterol and high blood pressure, intermittent fasting could lead to your dropping this medication.

While not proven in humans yet, intermittent fasting has shown impressive benefits in preventing cancer in animal studies. When these animals underwent intermittent fasting, they survived longer and had a reduction of symptoms from their tumors. Cancer is a disease that is not entirely understood and any research showing that this diet can help prevent it should be taken seriously. There was also a study that looked at humans going through chemotherapy. They found that the individuals who followed an intermittent fasting diet had fewer side effects from the chemotherapy. More research will need to be studied to understand fasting's relationship with cancer but so far it seems to be very positive.

There have many good effects shown throughout research on intermittent fasting but how does it work? How does intermittent fasting cause all these great benefits?

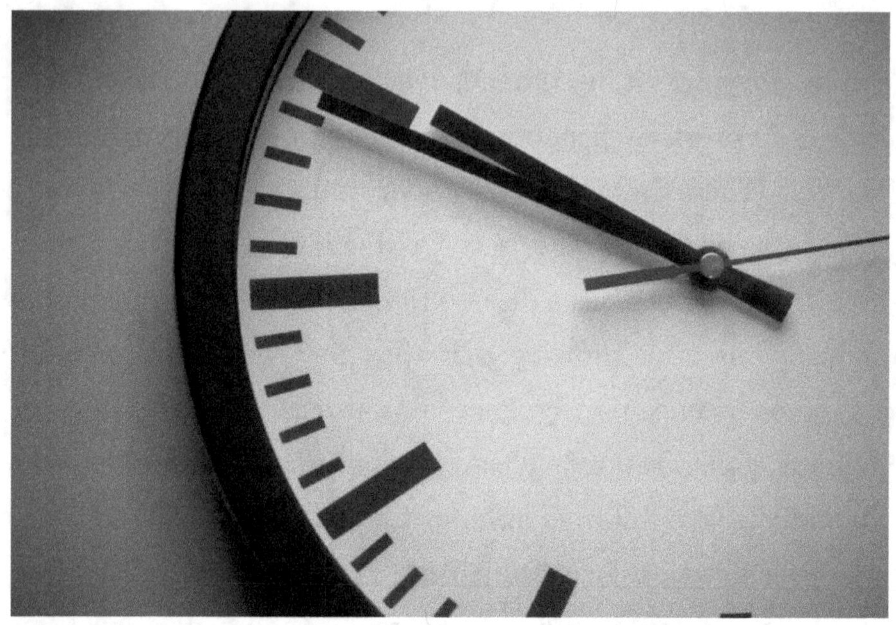

Just like calories from vegetables are better than calories from chocolate cake, the timing of meals consumption can affect how a human body stores it most efficiently. Usually, when we eat something, our metabolism spends hours burning through this food and digesting it. As the stomach digests this food, it will either use the energy or store the energy as fat. Hence, for someone constantly eating throughout the day, the body is going to use the nearest energy source. It is going to burn the calories of what was just eaten instead of the stored energy form body fat. It doesn't need body fat because it is constantly getting a new stream of energy from the food that is being consumed 3 or more times a day. With intermittent fasting, the body is not provided with consistent food at every few hour intervals. Hence, with the body realizing it is not receiving any food, it starts to burn the calories from stored energy, or fat cells. These fat cells become the only energy source available and therefore is being burned from body.

This can also happen if one workout while practicing intermittent fasting. During the process of fasting and post-workout, the body does not have sufficient glucose and glycogen to draw from due to meal skipped. So instead of burning through carbohydrates, where glucose and glycogen often come from, it is forced to look inward for energy. The easiest energy available is the fat stored in adipose tissue. This helps one to lose weight and become leaner. However, intermittent fasting does not stop there. It also aims to make one more sensitive to insulin. When we eat, our body produces insulin. Many individuals are becoming resistant to insulin because of frequent and short eating intervals on top of the high glycemic index food consumed. The more one eats, the more insulin that needs to be produced. While insulin is not inherently bad, if the person is not sensitive enough to insulin, he or she will never feel full and keep eating. Fasting changes how we produce and react to insulin. Due to of lesser amount of food consumed, our body is going to release less insulin. The more insulin sensitive one is, the better the body can store the calories consumed. When one breaks fast and starts eating, the body will either use up that energy immediately or store little of it, or it will be converted to glycogen and stored in muscles for use at a later time. Insulin is what is causing many people to gain weight. This insulin resistance is leading to overweight people and many different diseases. With intermittent fasting reducing insulin fluctuations and production, it creates a bunch of other great benefits.

Chapter 8: What You Need To Know About Hunger

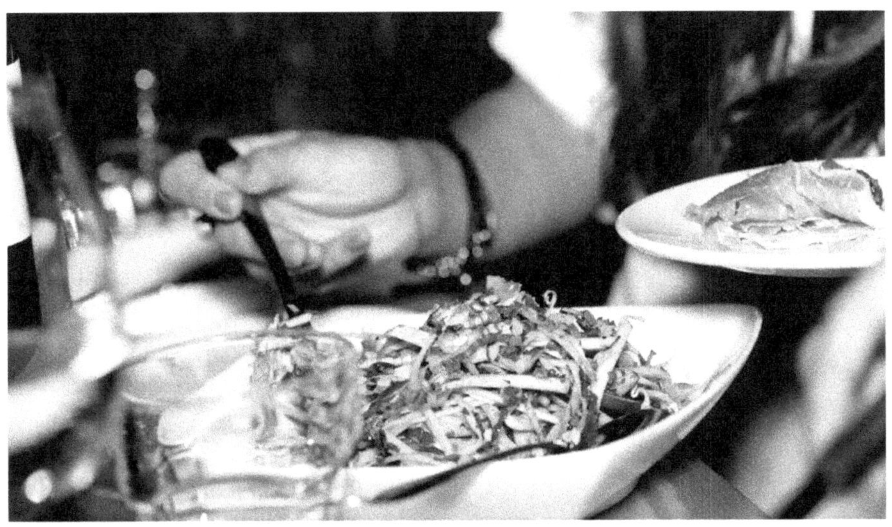

The biggest worry when someone starts thinking about intermittent fasting is how hungry he or she will be while fasting. First and foremost, hunger is different from food cravings. While hunger is necessary to ensure our survival, different chemicals in the brain cause food cravings. We can control food cravings. Many people find that they are viewing food cravings as hunger. When you start intermittent fasting, you may be hungry but you will also be hit with an onslaught of food cravings.

But, how does hunger work? Hunger begins with a hormone

being signaled in our brain. This hormone is termed as ghrelin. When our body finds that our blood sugar is low and our insulin levels are dropping, ghrelin signals the hypothalamus in the brain. Our brain is responsible for our basic body functions like when we are hungry or tired. The problem with this mechanism is that depends on other hormones to provide the signal. When insulin is dropping, it tells the brain that it needs food so it can spike back up again. Most people then eat something and insulin levels rise again. However, as mentioned in the previous chapter, insulin is what many people are becoming resistant to. That means more insulin needs to be released for one to feel hungry and full. Another chemical that works hand in hand with insulin is leptin. Leptin gets released from body's fat cells and trigger one to stop eating because body is already satisfied. The problem is that leptin and insulin are not instantaneous. They take a little while to be released. So many of us end up eating more than we need and then feel stuffed after our meal.

As mentioned before, hunger is different than food cravings. Our body does not constantly need food. In fact, it is not natural for our body to be constantly fed. We are not created to eat as often as we are now. In nature, food consumption is not at three times a day daily occurrence. Before civilization and urbanization, humans, food hunting is a daily human task. While we are at the top of the food chain, we are still inherently 'animals' scientifically. The only reason we feel like we are constantly hungry is due to changes in our insulin and leptin levels. These are the enemies indeed.

When we are hungry, Neuropeptide Y is released into our brain. The interesting thing is this tachykinin is also released when we are upset and angry. Have you ever been so hungry that you start to get mad? That is because the chemicals in your body are telling your brain over and over that they need food. Neuropeptide Y gets released and if we do not get food immediately, we can become angry suddenly. The reverse can also be true. When we get frustrated or upset, we tend to turn to food as remedy. These chemicals are running our hunger train. Therefore, there is an adjustment period for most when starting to embark on this intermittent fasting. It is almost certainly that one is going to feel hungry. But, much of this hunger is actually caused by food cravings, appetite or the habit of eating. Hence, our body does not need three meals a day. In fact, it could easily live off the fat stores and eat just three meals a week! While that is not the basis of intermittent fasting, one has to learn to manage such "feelings of hunger". No one wants to feel like they are starving all the time. Depending on the fasting method chosen, fluids can be drunk throughout the day. Drinking zero calorie drinks will help to remain in fasting state but can fill stomach up to trick brain into thinking it is getting food. If one is just starting intermittent fasting, it may be best to limit food but keep liquids in the diet to start.

Now, going back to hunger. It's all a trick. Human body is controlled by chemicals. These chemicals are causing our brain to be mad that they are not spiking every few hours. Thankfully, hunger is something that adapts. The more one does intermittent fasting, the more these chemicals and hormones are going to regulate. As fasting progresses, insulin and leptin levels will stabilize. What does this mean for hunger? It will get less frequent and less intense. They will not be begging for food constantly because they won't need to be replenished all the time. Ghrelin will not be released as often because insulin levels will not be spiking and dropping like they do when eating three meals a day. Since ghrelin is what controls hunger, once insulin levels stabilize, ghrelin will not notify the hypothalamus about hunger.

Hence, while one may feel hungry in the beginning of intermittent fasting, once the insulin levels have stabilized given some time, hunger pangs will be a thing of the past.

Chapter 9: The 6 Main Types of Intermittent Fasting

From the reading so far, you may think that fasting is absolutely not for you. The thought of skipping meals for a whole day seems like a crazy venture! Well, do not be alarmed. Fasting is surely not a one size fits all program. In fact, if anyone is asked to fast for 24 hours, highly likely he or she would decline too! Thankfully, intermittent fasting has multiple different methods you can try. One method is not necessarily better than the rest, you can just be sure that you will be able to find a method that works for you.

Generally, there are six different ways intermittent fasting can be done. These six different methods are 16/8 LeanGains, 5:2 diet, Eat Stop Eat, Alternate Day fasting, Warrior Diet, and Spontaneous Meal Skipping. Between all six methods you are bound to find a method that works for you. Some methods like the 16/8 method where you fast for 16 hours and eat for 8 hours, may be easiest for beginners. It should also be noted that women seem to have better success when their fast only lasts about 14 hours.

Because intermittent fasting has become so popular in the last few years, different forms of this beneficial diet have surfaced. If you already skip breakfast, you may find it easy to start up intermittent fasting. Throughout the next few chapters, more will be shared about each different method of intermittent fasting. You will then be able to decide which method may work best for you and learn the benefits of these different methods.

Chapter 10: 16/8 LeanGains Method

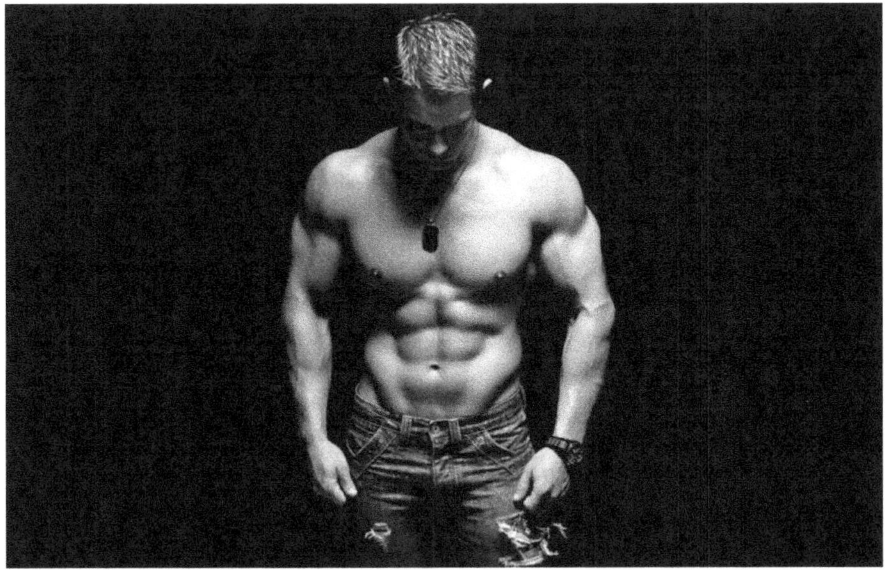

The first method to be described is called the 16/8 LeanGains Method. This method was developed by Martin Berkhan and he has became very popular for it. When most people think of intermittent fasting, this is the method that comes to their minds. So, what is this method?

The 16/8 LeanGains method is where you fast for 16 hours and eat all calories in an eight-hour window. Fasting for 16 hours may seem like a lot right off the bat, but there is only 24 hours in the day. If you are getting 8 hours sleep a night, that's only 8 hours throughout the day you need to fast. Yep, you read that right! Fasting during your sleep counts for this method! With this approach to intermittent fasting you are essentially just skipping breakfast. If you constantly wake up hungry, this may not be the best method for you. However, if you do not eat in the morning already, you are well on your way to intermittent fasting!

The most common way to practice this method is to break your fast at noon and stop eating at eight o'clock at night. That means that you eat all your calories from noon to 8PM and you fast from 8PM to noon. Moreover, , as you are probably sleeping from around 10PM to 6AM or 7AM, it is like you are only fasting from 8PM-10PM and 7AM-12PM. A lot of people really like this method because you do not have to skip full days of eating. If you stay busy while you fast, you hardly even know you are skipping breakfast!

Let's delve into this method a little more. What can you do and eat during your fast? You should not be eating or drinking any calories throughout your fasting period. If you want to drink black coffee with calorie free sweetener or 1 teaspoon of milk that is fine. You can also chew calorie free gum and drink whatever calorie free drinks you want to. So, if you cannot live without your diet soda, you will not have to. While calorie free gum and diet soda should always be had in moderation, if you need one of those during your fast period you may have it. You can also drink as much water as you need while you are fasting. Having sufficient water is crucial during fast as it aids in the brain function and detox process. While you are fasting, try to be productive. If you sit and wallow around the house, you are just going to feel hungry! Try to get as much done during your fasting window as possible.

When you break your fast, you can eat whatever meal you would like. It is recommended though that if you are not working out that day, that your first meal should be your largest. If you are working out, your post workout meal should be the largest. Therefore, if you work-out at 10AM and then decide to break your fast right after at 12PM, your first meal would be your largest. Consequently, if you work-out at 2PM, you should eat your largest meal right after your workout. However, if you decide to break your fast, just make sure that the timing is consistent. Our bodies' circadian clocks have to get used to routine. If we consistently break our fast at noon, but then break it at two another day, our body may become confused and start to feel hungry at odd times. Just try to stay consistent as to when your 8 hour window is.

This method is also great if you work night shifts or have an off schedule. You can choose to have your 8-hour window whenever you want. If you work late in the day, maybe you start your eating window at 3PM and go until 11PM. Whatever works for you. Just keep your eating window consistent.

Till this part you may feel that all sounds really great and may be wondering on the feedback or research studies so far. Thankfully, the LeanGains method has had some research studies done on it and there are many people who have tried this with huge success.

Many people argue that if you want to lose weight or gain muscle, eating at correct times is the recipe for success. They emphasize eating small (or big if trying to gain muscle) meals every 2-3 hours to keep metabolism going and put the calories needed into body. The supporters of intermittent fasting say that the timing of calories throughout the day does not matter for muscle gain. You can still eat three meals while doing the 16/8 LeanGains method. In fact, many studies have shown that users of this method are not losing muscle like some may think, they are just losing fat.

A study that watched individuals who were using the LeanGains method found that they lost three times the amount of fat as the individuals who followed a three meal a day protocol starting in the morning. Researchers attribute some of this fat loss to the fewer calories consumed by these individuals. What was interesting though was that this study also found that the chemical hormone adiponectin increased in the intermittent fasting group of individuals. What adiponectin does is that it convinces human brain to increase its energy expenditure. This means that the brain thinks it needs to burn more calories than it actually does. Thus, those doing intermittent fasting ended up burning more calories, therefore more fat loss. This is an incredible advantage to the LeanGains intermittent fasting. While both groups worked out the same amount of time with the same training per week, the adiponectin only increased in the intermittent fasting group. But, that is not all that happened. The intermittent fasting group also had their testosterone and IGF-1 levels decreased along with their insulin and blood sugar, cholesterol, and inflammation. The normal dieting group did not see any of these benefits. So, what do those indicators mean? All those levels will decrease when the body finds itself in a large caloric deficit. That is how one lose weight. However, the intermittent fasting group was not in a large enough caloric deficits to normally produce those results. So, in less scientific words, intermittent fasting can trick your body into thinking that it is eating fewer calories than it is which leads to more weight and fat loss. If you are looking at diet to lose weight, but hate diets, this 16/8 LeanGains method of intermittent fasting can help you attain the results you want. This method is also recommended for women because research has shown that women do better with shorter fasting periods. Are you one of those who hates counting calories and love having a daily routine? If so, this method may be best for you. The LeanGains method can be as easy as skipping breakfast and then going about your day as normal!

Chapter 11: The 5:2 diet

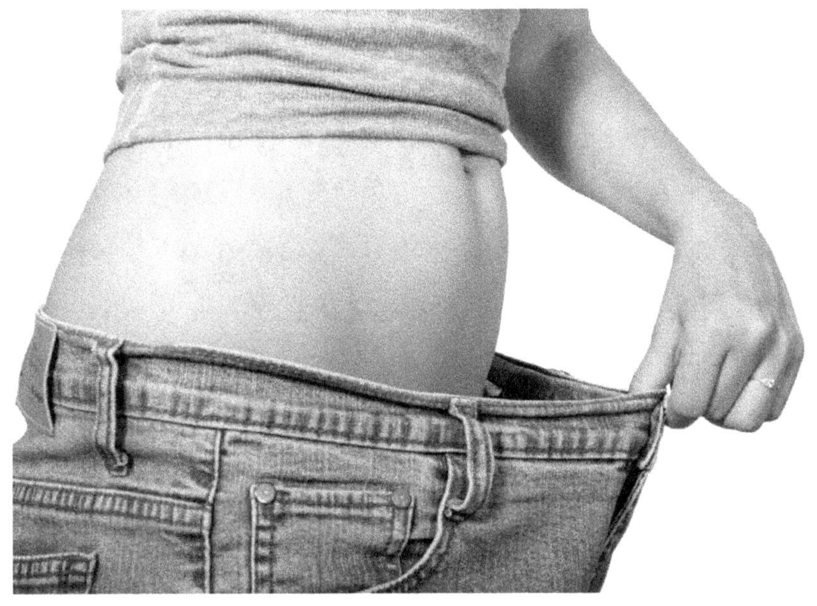

The 16/8 LeanGains diet might not be suitable for everyone. So, do not start thinking that intermittent fasting is not for you after just reading one method! There is literally a method for every kind of lifestyles for everyone. If you do not want to fast every day (even if it is only for 16 hours) then the 5:2 diet may be more of your style.

What is the 5:2 diet? The 5:2 diet is eating normally for 5 days and then restricting your calories on 2 days of the week. For 5 days, you eat 2000 calories for average women and 2400 calories for average men. On your two fast days you would eat 500 calories for average women and 600 calories for average men. The benefit that many people see in this diet is that they do not have to fast every day or alter too much of their daily routine. You only have to fast two days a week and the bonus is, you get to choose which two days you fast! Maybe you love weekends and cannot imagine fasting on a Friday or Saturday. Nobody's blaming you! Don't! Instead, choose to fast on Monday and Wednesday. Or if you do not want more stress on Mondays choose to fast on Tuesday or Thursday! You get to be in control of which days you fast on. The downside to this diet is that calories counting is required. While you can eat whatever you want up to the required calories on your non-fasting days, you still need to know how many calories you are consuming at each meal. Some people may go far beyond the required calories and not even realize it. To make sure that you are still at the required calories by monitoring the calories of your meal. The good thing about this is you do not have to skip out on something you want. If you want a piece of chocolate cake, eat the cake! Many people find that it is easy to stick to this diet when its only required to limit calories on some days. And the really nice thing with this diet is you never have to go a day without eating. On the two days that you fast, you are still eating a quarter of the calories you usually eat. If you cannot imagine skipping a day of eating or waiting to eat until the afternoon, this method of intermittent fasting may be best for you.

Research so far has been very positive about the 5:2 diet. Many animal studies have been done on this diet and found great benefits. A new study has recently come to light about the 5:2 diet on humans. This research followed a group of 100 overweight individuals. When compared to a group that restricted their calories on a daily basis, this group had lost much more weight. The 5:2 diet group lost up to 5 times more weight than the group who ate low calorie every day of the week. You may be thinking this sounds too good to be true. How does limiting your calories on two days turn out better than someone who limits their calories by less but does it every day of the week? The answer lies in the ease of this diet and insulin. The dieters who follow a 5:2 diet find that their insulin levels decrease. Many individuals who are often dieting have a problem with insulin resistance. Insulin resistance can cause massive weight gain and a feeling of never feeling full. When the individuals restricted their diet to 500 calories a day for two days a week, their insulin resistance got better. No longer did their body release insulin on such a huge scale. This in turn helped them to eat less every day of the week and heal their bodies from the overdose of insulin.

As with most intermittent fasting, the 5:2 diet also showed results in decreasing cholesterol levels and increasing metabolism speed. The 5:2 diet allows human body to heal faster. Whenever there is a heart attack or stroke in the animal studies, the brain repaired itself faster and avoided injury longer. This shows that the 5:2 diet is also good for helping overall brain and cardiovascular health.

This diet is beneficial for anyone who struggles with dieting. It is much easier to know that you only have to "diet" two out of 7 days of the week. Many people who have struggled with weight loss or dieting should consider this method as this method is best for people who want to lose weight but do not want to commit to a daily routine of fasting.

Chapter 12: Eat-Stop-Eat

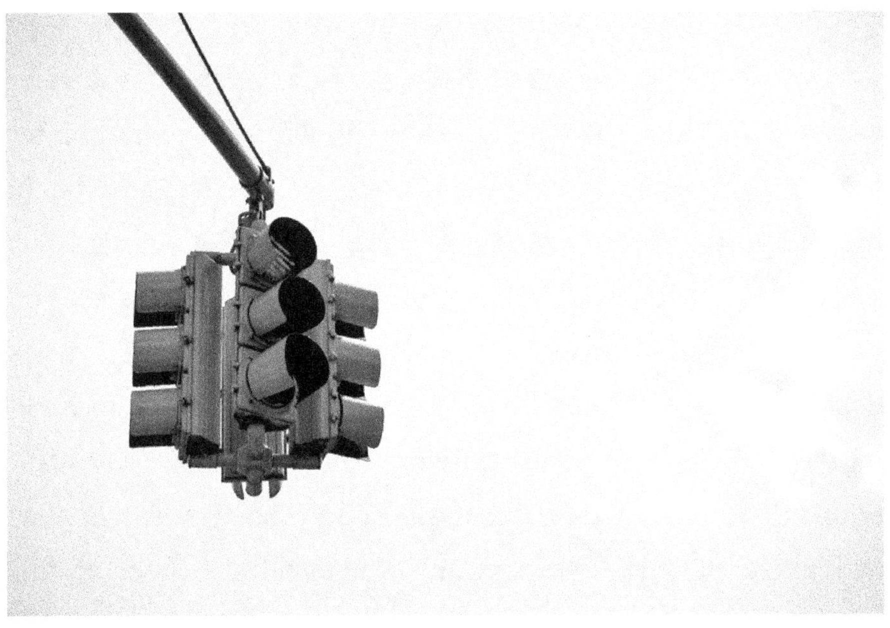

Next method here gets a little further into the fasting part of intermittent fasting. Some people do not like restricting their calories. They find themselves hungrier on days that they eat just a few calories than on days when they do not eat at all. This makes sense because when you eat, you start your metabolism. Hence, if you only eat 500-600 calories on your fast days, you may find yourself hungry. For this reason, many individuals find that they would rather fast for a full day with no calories at all. That is where the Eat-Stop-Eat diet comes into play.

The Eat-Stop-Eat diet was developed by a weight loss advisor named Brad Pilon. Brad Pilon came up with this method after finding that when individuals fasted, they seemed to be in better spirits, have more energy, and lose more weight. The Eat-Stop-Eat diet is very easy to follow. 5-6 days a week you will eat rather normally. Then on one or two days a week depending on your weight loss or health goal, you fast for a full 24 hours. This method extends your night fast by 8-10 hours. If you stopped eating at 8PM on Friday, you would start eating again at 8PM on Saturday. The benefit of choosing this fasting diet is that you only have to fast for one day a week. If you want greater results, you can fast for two days a week but you do not have to. If you do choose to fast for two days a week you need to choose two days that are separated by at least one day of eating. You should never be fasting for a full 48 hours. When you fast on this method, you break from food for a full 24 hours. If you cannot reach the 24 hours, you can limit your fast to 20 hours. During your fast, try to stay busy. You are able to work-out through your fast as you get used to it. You may find that you have more energy on your fasting days! You can and should continue to drink zero calorie fluids throughout the day. Most encouraged on this diet is to drink a lot of water. However, you can also drink dark coffee and other diet or zero calorie drinks. Ensuring sufficient water intake is important for body hydration.

Many individuals find this diet to be easiest for them because they get to eat normally on the other days of the week. What makes this different from the 5:2 diet is that on your fasting days you do not eat any calories. This may sound like a recipe to be miserably hungry but many people find that as they do not jumpstart their metabolism in the morning, their hunger stays satiated for a much longer time.

Well, one of the largest benefits to this diet is that researchers found that individuals who follow this method of intermittent fasting, do not binge eat the next day. You may think that if you fast for a full 24 hours then the next day you will be so ravenous to get food into your body that you will eat whatever you can get your hands on. Research has shown that it does not happen like that. While individuals often increase their calories the next day, it is usually only by about 10%. Therefore, a large caloric deficit is created by fasting for a whole day. Hence, you can lose weight much quicker with this large caloric deficit of about 2000 calories. Research also found that this method leads to more lean muscle mass gain. This is great for individuals who are trying to slim down but wants to maintain their muscle. Through this type of fasting, the cells become stressed and may perform better leading to anti-aging benefits. Studies also showed lower risk of chronic diseases while dieting with this method. Cholesterol is lowered and other hormones that lead to long-term health deterioration also decreased. And like the other methods of intermittent fasting, this also helps reduce the chance of insulin resistance. Insulin resistance is a serious problem, which can cause you to keep weight on and hold on to that stubborn stomach visceral fat.

While this method boasts lots of benefits, it does come with some trade-offs as well. Firstly, this diet is not for everyone. Because it is one of the more extreme intermittent fasting methods, only healthy individuals should try this method. Also, because of the lack of food for a full 24 hours many people may experience headaches or migraines when they first start out with this fasting method. While these side effects often go away after getting used to the fasting, some people report otherwise. This method also makes your social life rigid. If you have an event that day or friends invite you out for appetizers and drinks, you will not be able to eat anything. It is thus recommended to choose your fasting days wisely. It is also better to keep the same fasting days throughout the week so your body can count on the routine. Therefore, it is bound to interfere socially inevitably. Unlike the 5:2 diet, this diet does not tell you a calorie goal for the other days of the week so if you want to see results on the weighing scale, you will need to practice a lot of self-control.

Due to all these reasons, this diet might not suit everyone. If you are not new to intermittent fasting or you have fasted in the past and know how you react, this may then be a more suitable diet for you to consider. If you do not have large weight loss goals or just want to cut down on the amount of fat you have, the eat-stop-eat diet can help you to achieve these goals.

Chapter 13: Alternate Day Fasting

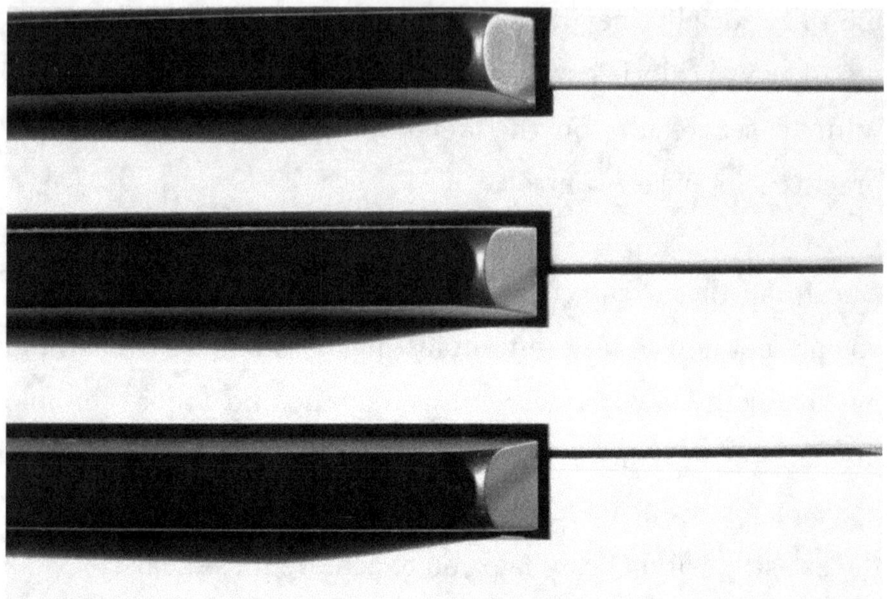

A similar approach to the Eat-Stop-Eat method, alternate day fasting provides attractive benefits too. The difference in alternate day fasting is that you are fasting every other day. While some people do indeed fast with no food, many take the same approach as the 5:2 diet and limit their calories on their fasting days to 500 calories. For example, with this diet you would fast Sunday, eat Monday, fast Tuesday, eat Wednesday, fast Thursday, eat Friday, fast Saturday, then eat on that next Sunday. So, some weeks you would fast four days and other weeks you would fast three days. Research has shown that if you limit your calories to 500 calories on your fasting days, it's just as effective as if you were doing a full day fast without any calories.

This diet approach to intermittent fasting is popular because it is easier than limiting your calories every day. But how is it easier? People do not like feeling deprived. When you have to limit your calories every single day you feel like you can never have what you want. However, with alternate day fasting you get to eat whatever you want on your non-fasting days. This way, you only need to restrict what you are eating half of the time. This allows people to think on their fasting days, "I want cake… Well I can always have it tomorrow." Instead of, "I hate dieting I just want cake." Traditional dieting has an incredibly high failure rate because people feel deprived and then give up their diet. With a non-diet approach, alternate day fasting allows you to eat what you want as long as it is on your non-fasting days. This diet is best for people who want to lose the most weight but do not want to fast without food for 24 hours.

Research has shown that alternate day fasting is especially beneficial for weight loss. With obese and overweight individuals losing up to 8% of their body weight in just weeks, this is a great non-diet approach. In addition to this, alternate day fasting has been shown to be superior to normal dieting at keeping muscle mass. When a calorie restrictive diet is attempted, weight loss is almost certain. But, most probably muscle mass will be reduced as well. This is part of the downside for traditional dieting. However, alternate day fasting has been shown to interestingly help increase muscle mass while providing larger fat loss as well. One benefit of alternate day fasting is that it works well with middle-aged men and women. Middle-aged individuals often have the hardest time losing weight. Because of this, they try many diets a year and often end up gaining more weight throughout their diet changes. Alternate day fasting has been shown to help even out hormones and promote a greater weight loss in middle-aged individuals.

Perhaps one of the best benefits that alternate day fasting can provide is the change it makes to your hunger. Studies have shown that some people believe their hunger to be less on the days they fast whereas others say it has not changed. What is most fascinating is that alternate day fasting decreases lepton and ghrelin. Leptin is a hormone released by our adipose tissue that signals our brain that we are full. Ghrelin is the opposite and is released when our body signals it needs more energy or calories. When leptin thresholds are high, more food will be required to give the full feeling. When ghrelin levels are high one tends to eat more in calories and more often than needed. Alternate day fasting lowers these levels. What this means is you will take less food to get full and you will feel hungry less often. This is a benefit for anyone who finds themselves feeling hungry and never getting full. Alternate day fasting can help reset your hunger chemicals so that you are not overeating which consequently causes the weight gain. As such, this is a great way to do intermittent fasting. While some people may have a hard time sticking to under 500 calories every day, the benefits often outweigh the cons.

Another reason why alternate day fasting is popular and beneficial is the way it affects metabolism. When calories are restricted on a normal diet, metabolism slows down. When metabolism slows down, more fat tends to be stored in the body from the food consumed. Therefore, this explains why so many diets end up failing. While one is on diet, metabolism is actually wrecked. Research has shown that alternate day fasting does not affect metabolism in any significant way. Hence, while calories are restricted, metabolism is not wrecked.

If you are not looking to lose weight, alternate day fasting can still be helpful for your health. In normal weight individuals, studies have found that following alternate day fasting reduced their fat mass and increased their fat burning. Their insulin lowered too. Therefore, if you are already at your desired weight but looking to reduce your body fat, alternate day fasting can help you with this goal.

So who is this fasting method best for?
Alternate day fasting is suitable quite a wide range of people with different needs. If you are in middle age and wants to lose a lot of weight, this is a great option. You only have to restrict what you eat half of the time and you can get all the benefits of a normal calorie restriction diet. If you are in the middle of your training season, this is also a good fasting method for you. Alternate day fasting does not necessarily cut down on your muscle mass (with sufficient calorie intake) but increase the amount of fat burn. So, if you need to burn fat quickly then this method can help you keep your muscle and get you leaner.

Because you are restricting your diet to only 500 calories every other day, you need to eat nutritious food for your body on the days you are fasting. If you try to eat junk food on fasting day, you are going to hit your 500-calorie limit a lot faster. In order to keep your hunger at bay and still stay under 500 calories, try to eat a lot of lean protein on fasting days.

Chapter 14: The Warrior Diet

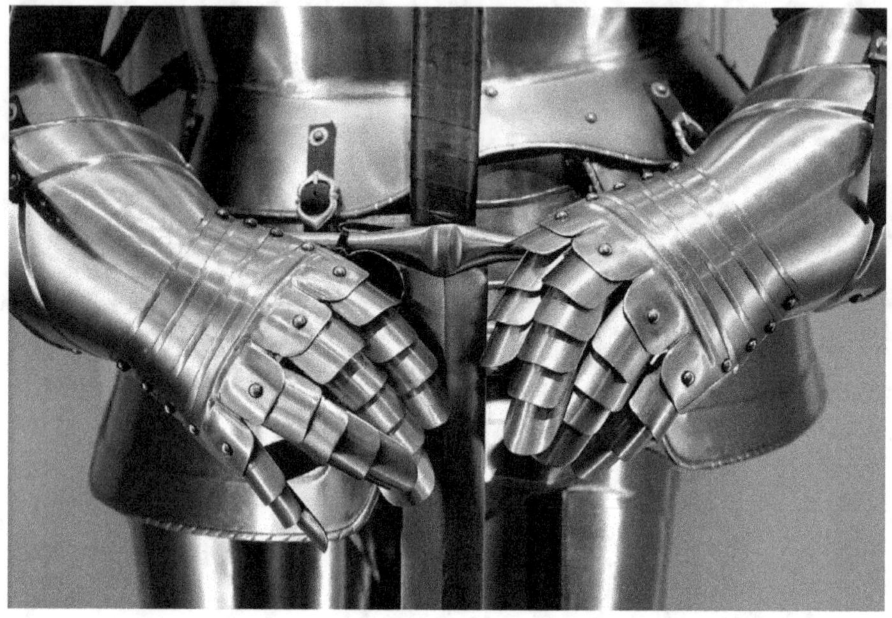

The warrior diet was developed almost 20 years ago by Ori Hofmekler. While still a form of intermittent fasting, the warrior diet focuses on recreating the natural way our ancestors used to eat. The basis of it is to eat very few calories throughout the day and then have one big meal at night. They call your daytime eating "under eating" because you only eat a few calories throughout the day. You can eat small servings of fresh fruit and vegetables, nuts and seeds, and other non-processed foods. You can also fast from liquids throughout the day but if you feel you cannot handle that, you can have non-calorie drinks like water, coffee, and tea. The basis of this diet is taken from what warriors used to eat in armies like Ancient Rome and Sparta. If you were a warrior, you would not have time to eat much during the day because you would be hunting for your food for the night or fighting as an army. As such, ancient warriors would eat one large meal (their "hunt") when night fell upon them. This diet believes that our bodies are made to be nocturnal eaters, eating our largest meal at dark. This diet also says that you should be exercising on an empty stomach for best results. While following the warrior diet, you do not count calories. Your sole focus is getting that nightly meal and eating as much as you can, essentially force feeding yourself a large enough meal to account for the calories you need for the day.

This diet is one of the more extreme versions of intermittent fasting but also one of the earliest versions developed. As it does not consider that not everyone is used to fasting every day until one late meal, the warrior diet requires a greater adjustment period. It is recommended to start with 2-3 days a week of the warrior diet until your body gets used to not having 3 full meals and snacks throughout the day.

Unfortunately, even though the warrior diet has been around

for quite some time, there is not much extensive research done on this eating method. In fact, it is one of the least researched methods of intermittent fasting. The warrior diet makes some big claims about how eating one meal a day is what our body is created for. However, there is a lack of science backing that this is true.

One of the largest things the warrior diet has going for it is that it talks about healthy eating. A lot of the other intermittent fasting methods are not based on nutrition. They are mostly based on the timing of the meal. While this can still yield results, eating healthier can allow you to achieve your desired healthy body faster and it is never bad to fill your body with healthy nutrients. The large meals you eat at night as well as the fasting snacks you can have during the day are all healthy. Focus will be on protein and healthy fats in addition to fruits and vegetables. In addition to healthy eating, this is still a form of intermittent fasting. Since intermittent fasting has been studied extensively, you can assume that this diet will lead to the same success other methods of intermittent fasting have showed.

Among the few studies done on the warrior diet, one was researched about how the warrior diet affects muscle mass and fat. Based on name alone, most people would assume that this diet is for people who want to gain muscle and become large hulking warriors. Well, part of that assumption may be true. The research found that when an individual ate the one large meal at night, they lost more fat and gained more muscle. This warrior diet group was compared with a group of individuals who ate three meals a day. The interesting part of this research is that both groups were consuming the same number of calories, and yet the warrior diet came out ahead for weight loss and muscle gain. This study also found however that leptin and ghrelin increased throughout the study and the warrior diet group became hungrier. This means that their hormones did not adapt to the diet. This is something to think about when starting this diet; you may still be hungry throughout the day with no food in sight until the evening. Another important thing to mention is that it may be hard to get all the nutrients you need just in one meal. Because of this, proprietors of the warrior diet say you should be taking an all-natural multivitamin to ensure you are getting the nutrients your body will need.

Regardless of the lack of scientific evidence, there are thousands of personal accounts of people who have made the warrior diet work for them. Just like it's cool name, this diet is obviously not for the weak of heart. If you are planning on trying to gain muscle but you do not want to gain fat in the process, this may be the intermittent fasting diet for you. This diet could also work for busy individuals who may only have time for one meal anyhow. Or, this diet may be best to be altered to a few times a week and then eating normally on the other days. If pigging out at one-meal sounds like your type of diet, you may want to give this one a try.

Chapter 15: Spontaneous Meal Skipping

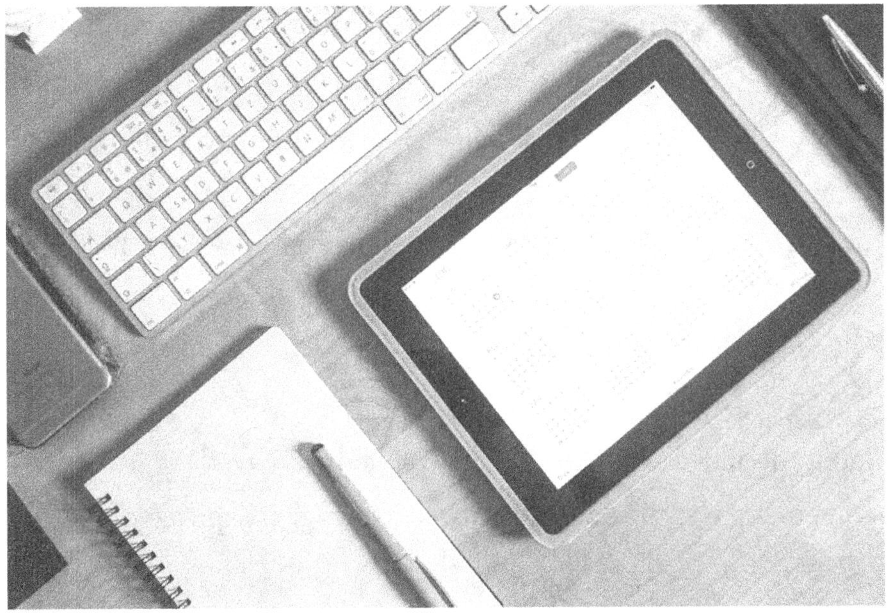

How many times have you been too busy to eat and you skip lunch? Or when you are running late, you rush out the door without breakfast? Well, guess what? You just practiced spontaneous meal skipping! If you are someone who likes to dip your toes in before you take the plunge, spontaneous meal skipping will be your preferred intermittent fasting method. Spontaneous meal skipping doesn't really have a creator, its basis lies in eating when you are hungry, and skipping a meal when you are not hungry. You do not plan it out; you learn to listen to your body. If you are used to eating 3 meals and snacks in between, it can be hard to listen to your hunger signals on this method of intermittent fasting. Most likely, your hunger chemicals will be high because of how you have previously eaten. Therefore, it will be hard to spontaneously skip meals because you will probably be hungry for every meal. If this is the case, you may need to spend the first few days planning your skipped meal before you can start listening to your body and spontaneously skipping meals.

Spontaneous meal skipping is typically viewed as the most convenient way to do intermittent fasting. If you have a social event or dinner sprung upon you, you don't have to fast! You can decide to fast for a different meal and change up your routine. Spontaneous meal skipping does not require you to have any routine. This way you can be spontaneous throughout your fasting routine. A lot of people like this approach because it does not require a big lifestyle change. Some of the other forms of intermittent fasting require dedication to a routine so that your body will get used to the rhythm. Spontaneous meal skipping is the opposite. This form of intermittent fasting relies on surprising your body and choosing to skip different meals. You end up getting an easy to follow diet and because you are restricting calories, you will lose weight as well. People have an easier time choosing this diet because they get to decide whenever they want to fast. However, this can also be a bad thing. If you do not have a lot of self-control when it comes to dieting, this form of intermittent fasting might not be the best for you. If you do not choose to skip your meals often, this diet is not going to be effective for you. You may find this diet to be very hard if you do not have strong willpower.

The science behind this method is quite interesting and sound. However, this method only works if you do not eat more at your next meal. Research has shown that if you eat just as many calories at your next meal as you should have had at the meal you skipped, your insulin and glucose actually rise. These in turn make you hungrier and keep weight on. However, if you skip your meal and then do not eat more at your next meal, you will find yourself with all the benefits of intermittent fasting like lower cholesterol, less fat mass, and weight reduction. This is one of the only methods that can negatively affect your health if you eat more at your next meal. That means that you need to be aware of what you are eating and how many calories you are eating at your next meal.

So who is this diet best for? Busy people can benefit a lot from this type of intermittent fasting. You do not have to plan when you fast and you can fast for breakfast, lunch, or dinner. If you really want breakfast one day and the next day you really don't want lunch, you can eat breakfast and skip lunch and then eat at dinner time! This diet is good for teaching people to listen to their body. If you are already at your weight goal, this can be a good diet for you too. This can help you to reset your hunger hormones and allow you to tune into your body and learn how to tell if you are truly hungry or not. This diet is best for people with strong willpower because there is not a plan in place. You must be okay with spontaneity and allow yourself the opportunity to be relaxed about which meals you eat versus skip.

Chapter 16: How to break your fast

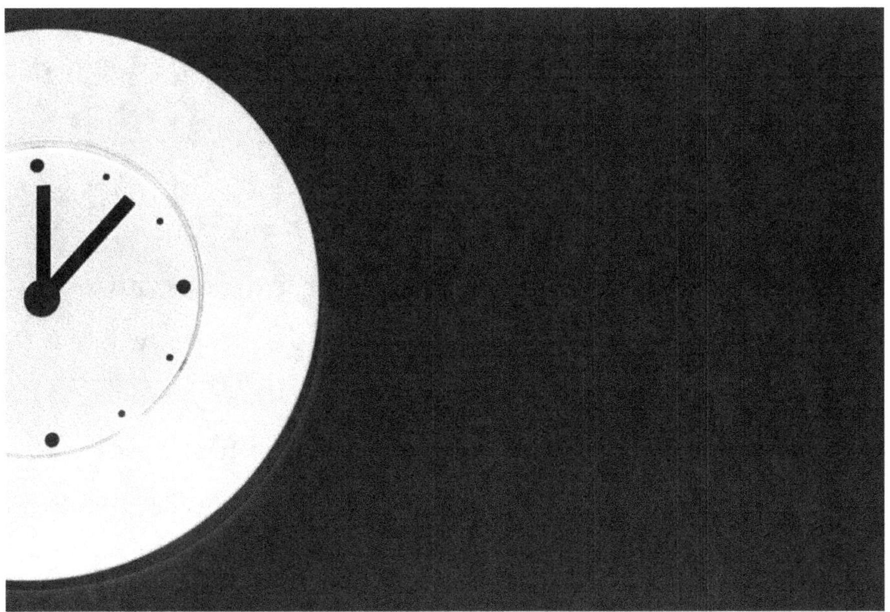

When you practice intermittent fasting, regardless of the fasting methods used, you will have to break your fast at some point. While with some methods it may not matter as much how you break your fast, other methods you must be careful on how you break your fast. The longer you fast, the more cautious you should be about breaking your fast. If you want to work out in your fasting state, which some research says this can help you to gain more muscle mass, then you should not break your fast until you are done working out. Once you break your fast, your post-work out meal should be your largest meal. You should break your fast whenever your method you choose says so. For example with the warrior diet, you would break your fast at night with one large meal. With the 5:2 diet, you would not break your fast until the morning of one of your non-fast days.

But, with all these said, what should you break your fast with? If you are fasting fluids, try to break your fast first with a glass of water. Before you eat food, it is important to get water into your system so that you are not eating more than you need to be eating. It is always best to break your fast with just water and instead of other fluid. While diet sodas and other non-calorie drinks are often allowed on different methods of intermittent fasting, you may want to avoid them. These drinks that contain zero calorie sweeteners can cause you to crave more sugar and subsequently gain weight. In addition to these effects, research has linked artificial sweeteners with a large variety of health issues including food allergies, weight gain, hormonal imbalances, and even cancer. When you cut these artificial sweeteners out of your diet, you will start to crave less sugar. This is obviously beneficial because sugar is what causes our insulin to spike and can lead to insulin resistance and weight gain. Therefore, if you want to get healthier, you should be choosing water, unsweetened teas, and unsweetened coffee as your choice of fluid. It is especially important to drink as much water as you can since water is essential for the detoxification process and also helps to deliver oxygen throughout the body with added function of regulating body temperature.

Once you have had your glass of water, what should you be eating to break your fast? While many of these diets do not specify what you should eat on your non-dieting days, it is important to still watch what you eat. Sure, you may be able to get some of the benefits of intermittent fasting if you fast on fasting days and then eat whatever you want on your non-fasting days. However, is all that junk food beneficial to your body? If you want to be healthy and give your body the best benefits that intermittent fasting has to offer, you need to watch what you eat. Most of the intermittent fasting methods do not require you to watch what you eat nor do they tell you to count your calories on your non-fasting days. In reality, you probably do not need to count your calories since you have created such a large caloric deficit with your fasting days. However, if you want to lose fat and gain muscle, you need to eat a lot of protein, healthy fats, and whole foods like fruits and vegetables. You should be able to eat enough of these items to feel satiated but not overly full. If you stuff yourself full for every meal on your non-fasting days then you are not going to feel well and your body will not be at its healthy peak form.

It is recommended to break your fast with something high in protein and healthy fat. Something like grilled chicken with avocado and fresh roasted vegetables. If you want to break your fast with a snack, break it with something like nuts and carrots or an apple with all-natural almond or peanut butter. Whether you break your fast with a meal or snack depends on what intermittent fasting method you are following. Some people like to break their fast with a snack so that they are not putting so much food into their stomach all at once. Sometimes, when you eat too big of a meal quickly, you may end up feeling nauseous. If you have this problem, try breaking your fast with a small snack first.

Chapter 17: Have a Plan in Place

Maybe the most important part of intermittent fasting is having an action plan in place. Besides spontaneous meal skipping, which doesn't require a plan, all other forms of intermittent fasting should have an action plan. You should be planning the days you fast, what you will be eating on your fast days (if allowed), and what you will be eating on your non-fast days. If you are truly trying to take on intermittent fasting and looking to get healthier, you will need to plan so that you have healthy foods available to you always.

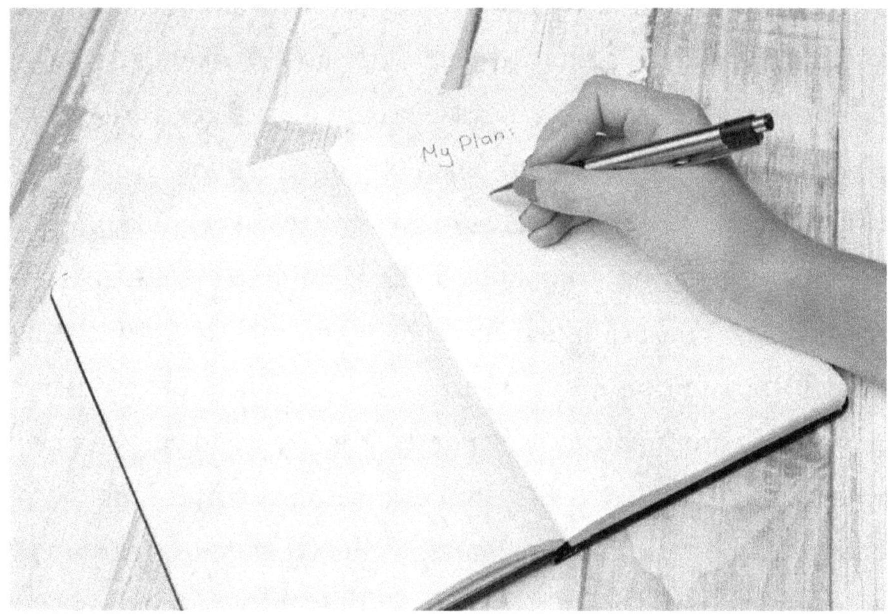

How do you create a plan? Get out your planner or your calendar. You can even just make a note on your phone or plan everything out on your phone calendar. You could even download and use any of the intermittent fasting apps available on handphone to help you plan.

First, you need to schedule when you will be fasting. If you are planning on following spontaneous meal planning, you will not need to plan it specifically. Feel free to skip this chapter. To plan your fasting days, go over your weekly schedule. You should want your fasting days to fall on a day where you are not too busy and are unlikely to be out with friends. For example, if you and your friends typically go out for drinks on Fridays, you should not choose Friday as a fasting day. Weekends are also often not suitable fasting days because people tend to go out and dine with family and friends on weekends. Take into consideration your work schedule, your social schedule, and all activities including your spouse and children's schedules (if applicable). You are much more likely to stick to your fasting days if they fall on a day where there are not a lot of outside temptations to break your fast early. Hence, try to choose a day where there will not be office meetings with doughnuts, children's performances or games, and other tempting day to day items. It can also help to plan your fasting days on days that you need to get a lot done. If you find yourself working the longest on Wednesdays, Wednesday may be a good fasting day. When you are not focused on your next meal, you become a lot more productive. In addition to that, if you are super busy throughout the day you will find yourself focusing less on food and may not even notice you are fasting! Anything to help curb your thoughts of food is a good thing. Thus, when choosing your fasting days, keep your business and productivity in mind.

The next thing to plan is what you will be eating on the days you are fasting. If you fast completely without food, this will not apply to you. However, some diets like the 5:2, the warrior diet, and alternate day fasting require you to fast but still eat around 500 calories. While 500 calories may seem like a lot, those calories can go rather quickly depending on what you eat. You could have a full cup of broccoli for 30 calories or you could have an apple with a fourth of a cup of peanut butter and eat about 400 calories. While an apple and peanut butter are a healthy snack on a non-fasting day, it can be detrimental to your calorie count on a fasting day. Since you need to keep your calorie count low, you need to watch what you eat on your non-fasting days.

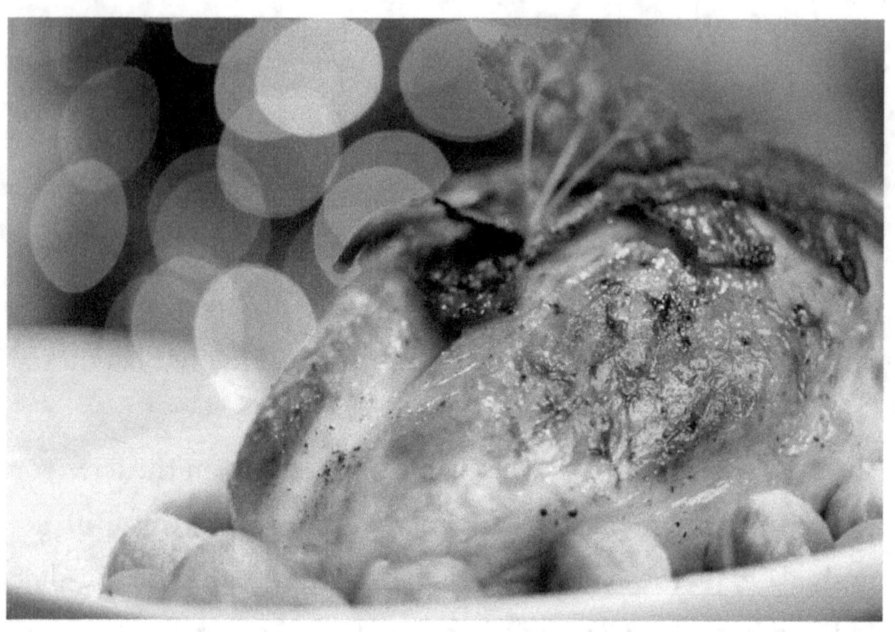

Try to eat things with lean protein to keep you full longer. Food like chicken breast, roasted vegetables and fruit, and small amounts of fat will help you to still feel satiated while fasting but not ruin your calorie count. Therefore, it is so important to have a plan for your fasting days. If you do not plan your snacks and meals, you can end up eating too much or you may end up not being able to eat anything at all! If you do not have already made snacks prepared throughout the day, you will be more likely to reach out for fast food. Not only will this food be high in calories and unhealthy, it also will not keep you full. You will end up eating these fast food items to find that you are hungry a mere hour later. Can you imagine fasting throughout the day and being hungry all day because you chose to eat some French fries instead of a healthy snack? You will be miserably hungry and give up fasting! Making yourself have a plan will allow you to enjoy intermittent fasting. If you enjoy intermittent fasting, you are going to do it longer and your health will benefit more.

If you are doing intermittent fasting you are either trying to lose weight or get healthier. In order to achieve either, you need to watch what you eat when you are not fasting as well. If you eat junk food every day except for your fasting days, what will happen? Well, you may still benefit some from intermittent fasting but your body will not become much healthier. You may not lose weight nearly as fast if you choose to eat unhealthy on those days. So, what does healthy eating have to do with having an action plan? It has everything to do with having an action plan! If you want to look better and feel better, you need to eat healthy. If you want to make healthy eating easier, you need to meal plan.

Now that does not mean you need to make every meal in advance, but it does mean that you need to think ahead where and what you are going to be eating. If you are hungry at work and did not pack a lunch, what are your options? Restaurant food or fast food. While you may try to argue that restaurant food can be healthy, it is fairly challenging to make that a reality. You see, even if you order a salad at a restaurant, with the toppings and dressing, you are loading your plate with unhealthy fat and sodium. Fast food and restaurant food are notoriously high in sodium. As sodium is linked to a bunch of issues like high blood pressure, it is best to keep your sodium intake down. That is nearly impossible if you are constantly eating out. If you are going to be away from home for a snack or a meal, bring something with you. Not only will you save money by not eating out as much, you will also be getting a much more healthy and nutritious meal.

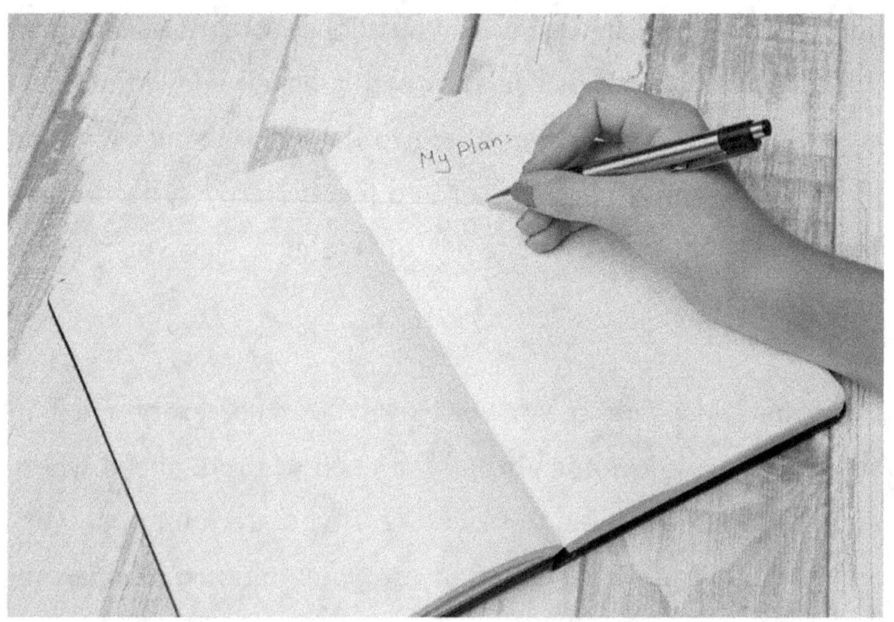

Eventually if you do not plan your meals and snacks on fasting and non-fasting days, you could be setting yourself up for failure. Intermittent fasting can be a hard protocol to follow and if you do not plan well, it becomes even more difficult. Failing to plan will make you grow tired of intermittent fasting. It is much easier to plan and make your intermittent fasting experience happier and easier!

Chapter 18: Fasting Fluids

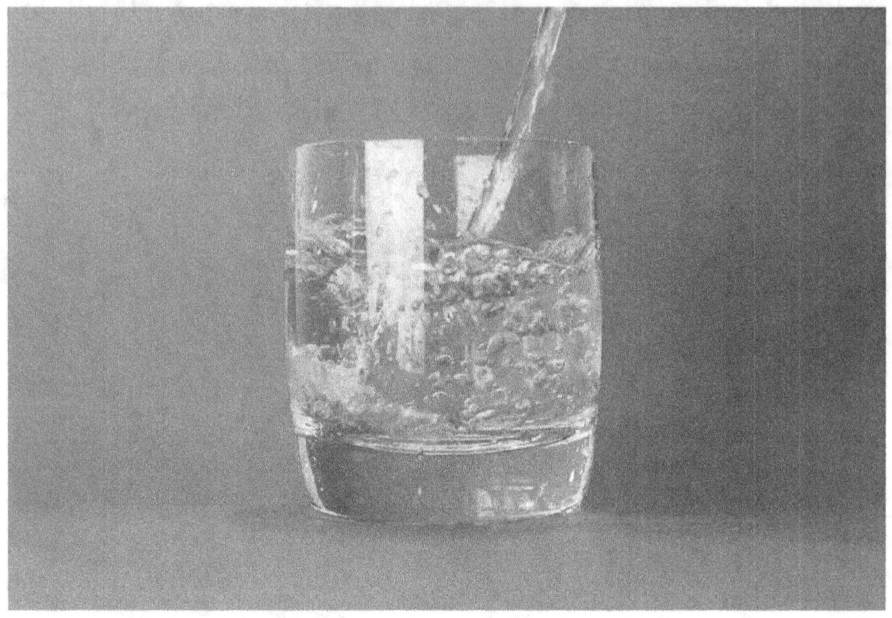

One of the grey areas of intermittent fasting is your fluid intake. This is when you do not drink anything in addition to not eating anything. Or, it can also be limiting your fluids to liquids that contain less than 50 calories throughout the day. If you fast from fluids completely, this should never be done longer than a one-day period. While fasting from all fluids may be something familiar to body builder before a competition, it is not exactly all that healthy for you. Our bodies run on water. While we can live for a few weeks without a reliable food source, we would die within a few days if we did not have water. Our cells and plasma are made up of water. Therefore, it is so important to make sure we are drinking sufficiently throughout the day. Our body needs water to function.

Nonetheless, there are some reasons that people fast completely from all fluids. One reason may be for religious fasting. Many religions ask that you fast from food and drink for a certain amount of time. They believe that when you turn your focus away from food and drink then you are more open for spiritual progression. Some individuals also apply this to productivity and a detox of the diet. They say that by taking your focus away from food and drink, your body can detox itself and focus more on the regeneration of cells and it helps to restart your hormones and metabolism. If taking this approach, just remember not to do it very often and definitely not longer than a day. Another reason some may want to fast from liquids is due to specific body building regime. Before body building competitions, competitors will start to fast from liquids the day before. While water can be an important weight loss tool, it does add weight when you first consume it. This is why body builders refrain from water the day before competitions, they do not want to look bloated or have any extra weight.

A more popular approach to fasting fluids is to cut out any

fluids with calories. Drinks that have calories like sodas and juices do not provide you with adequate amounts of energy. These drinks are called "empty calories." Empty calories cause you to put on weight but give no added benefit. Think of it like this. How many times have you had a soda at an event? Even though you just filled your body with one hundred and fifty plus calories, you are still hungry. If you would have eaten the same amount of calories in the form of chicken or broccoli, you would be satisfied for a while. Hence, you should fast from calorie filled drinks. Many people put on weight because they drink copious amounts of soda. While it may give you some caffeine and you like the flavor, it does not give your body the nutrients it needs to survive and thrive.

If you want to do intermittent fasting correctly, you will need to fast from fluids that contain calories. We recommend drinking large amounts of water with some coffee or tea. While you can have diet soda since it contains no calories, we do not recommend it. In fact, diet sodas can be more harmful to your health because they contain artificial sweeteners. These artificial sweeteners have been linked to a host of problems including weight gain and cancer. They also make you crave sugar more. So, if you want to do intermittent fasting the best possible way, try to stick to water.

The general rule of intermittent fasting is that if your drinks contain less than 50 calories, your body will then remain in the fasting state. But this does not mean you should add 50 calories worth of sugar into your drink. What this means is that you can have a splash of milk in your coffee or a lemon slice or other pieces of fruit in your water. Just watch out for high amounts of sugar and caffeine. Your main drink should always be water but if you cannot give up your coffee and tea, those are acceptable a few times throughout the day. If you are sick of water, try exploring naturally flavored seltzer waters. The carbonation can give you that soda effect but they are just sparkling water and contain no calories.

Chapter 19: Bonus! Snack Recipes

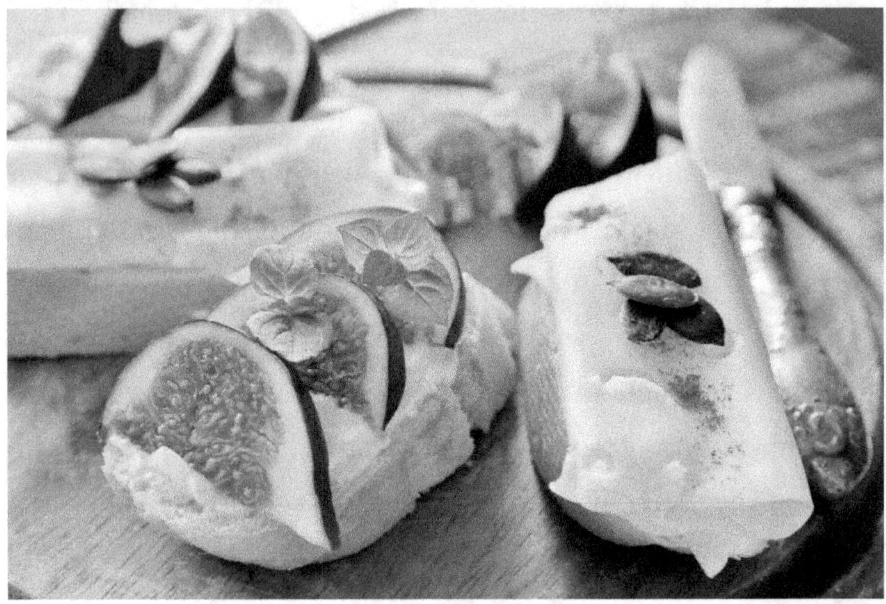

It is totally understandable that we may get a sudden hunger pangs at times where we least expect it. This is particularly so important to have the right healthy snacks prepared when such times come. Hence, this section is written for the exact purpose of equipping you with some simple snack recipes for such handy hungry moments!

Egg Cups

Serving Size: 1 muffins | Prep Time: 10 minutes | Cook Time: 20 minutes
Nutritional Info:
Calories per muffin: 62, Fat: 3.2 g, Protein: 5 g, Carb: 5.5 g

This is the easiest snack to have on your fasting days. It is filled with protein, has little calories, and will make sure you remain full. These egg cups are easy to prepare and keep well in the fridge for a week. You can choose to heat them up in the microwave or keep them cold. They taste great either way!

Ingredients:

6 large eggs

1/2 tsp sea salt

1 cup shredded cheese

1 cup packed spinach

6 pieces bacon, cooked and crumbled

Directions:

1. Preheat the oven to 350 F. Grease your muffin tins with non-stick spray.

2. Crack your eggs into a bowl and mix well. Add in your shredded cheese, spinach, bacon and salt and stir to combine.

3. Spoon the mixture into 12 muffins tins.

4. Bake in preheated oven for 20-22 minutes.

Kale Chips

Serving Size: 1/6 recipe| Prep Time: 10 minutes | Cook Time: 10 minutes
Nutritional Info:
Calories per servings: 58, Fat: 2.8 g, Protein: 2.5 g, Carb: 7.5 g

Everyone has that craving for something salty. Instead of reaching for the nearest bag of chips, think about whether it is going to help you stay satisfied throughout the day. Most likely, it will not! Save yourself the grease and calories and make these kale chips. Not only do they satisfy that crunchy and salty craving, they are also a great source of much-needed vitamins and minerals throughout your fasting routine. If you want to try mixing it up, you can season these with your favorite seasoning salt instead of sea salt. If you like things spicy, add a little bit of cayenne pepper on top!

Ingredients:

1 large bunch of kale

1 tsp sea salt

1 Tbs extra virgin olive oil

Directions:

1. Preheat the oven to 350 F.

2. Remove the leaves from the thick stems. Break each leaf

into chip sized pieces.

3. Place kale into a bowl and toss with olive oil and sea salt.

4. Place onto a cookie sheet lined with foil or parchment paper.

5. Bake in the oven for approximately 10 minutes and edges are browned.

Celery Fruit Sticks

Serving Size: 1 celery stalk | Prep Time: 10 minutes | Cook Time: 0 minutes
Nutritional Info:
Calories per serving: 91, Fat: 6 g, Protein: 5 g, Carb: 6.5 g

If you need an easy to prepare snack that will keep well in your lunch, these celery fruit sticks are the winner. These are super easy to prepare in the morning. They pack well in any lunch and the protein and healthy fats will help to curb your hunger and keep you satisfied even on your hungriest days. Do not be tempted by your coworkers junk food snacks, this snack will leave you feeling great and is absolutely delicious!

Ingredients:

5 stalks of celery

½ cup natural unsweetened peanut butter

½ cup unsweetened raisins

Directions:

1. Cut your celery stalks in half.
2. With a knife or spreader, spread the inside of the celery stalk with peanut butter.
3. Take your raisins and line the peanut butter covered celery stalk with a line of raisins.

4. Eat and enjoy!

Homemade Granola Bars

Serving Size: 1 bar | Prep Time: 10 minutes | Cook Time: 35 minutes
Nutritional Info:
Calories per bar: 162, Fat: 5.2 g, Protein: 3 g, Carb: 20 g

Sometimes, you just want a snack that reminds you of those unhealthy snack aisles at the store. These granola bars taste great but are not filled with the preservatives and chemicals that are often in all of the grocery store snacks. While this snack is slightly higher in calories, the oats will help to keep you full. This is also a great snack for non-fasting days because this recipe makes 24 servings! It is easy to grab one of these as you walk out the door in the morning. After you try this recipe, you will not be missing those bars from the grocery store. In fact, this recipe will not only wow your taste buds, but everyone is your family's taste buds as well!

Ingredients:

2 cups rolled oats

½ cup honey

½ cup wheat germ

¾ tsp cinnamon

1 cup flour

¾ cup unsweetened raisins

¾ tsp salt

1 egg

½ cup coconut oil

2 tsp vanilla extract

¾ cup coconut sugar

Directions:

1. Preheat your oven to 350 F.
2. Spray a 9 x 13 baking dish with non-stick spray
3. Combine all ingredients into a large mixing bowl and mix well.
4. Spread evenly into prepared baking dish
5. Cook for 35 minutes or until the top looks golden brown
6. Cool in the pan for five minutes and then cut them into 24 bars.

Spicy Jicama

Serving Size: ¼ recipe | Prep Time: 10 minutes | Cook Time: 0 minutes
Nutritional Info:
Calories: 77, Fat: 0.7 g, Protein: 1.7 g, Carb: 17 g

If you have not tried jicama, get ready for a super yummy vegetable. This veggie often is forgotten about in the grocery store shelves. But, it is not for good reason! When you dress up jicama with a little bit of lime and spice you will find yourself craving more! This crunchy veggie will make you forget about the chips your coworker is munching on. This recipe is low in calories and requires zero cook time! It is easy to prepare and is easy to make last minute if you forget to make a snack the night before.

Ingredients:

1 large jicama

2 Tbs lime juice

2 Tbs Chili powder

½ tsp cayenne pepper

Directions:

1. Peel and slice your jicama into bite size 1-inch pieces.

2. In a medium bowl, toss with lime juice, chili powder, and

cayenne pepper.

3. Separate into four servings and serve.

Fresh Salsa

Serving Size: 1/16 recipe | Prep Time: 10 minutes | Cook Time: 0 minutes
Nutritional Info:
Calories: 15, Fat: 0 g, Protein: 0.5 g, Carb: 3 g

Who does not love salsa? Salsa is so delicious! Are you stuck dreaming of the chips and salsa at your favorite Mexican restaurant? Eating the chips and salsa at your favorite restaurant can amount to almost double your daily fasting intake. To ensure your calories are kept under 500 on a fasting day, ditch your restaurant and make your own salsa at home. This recipe is incredibly easy and amazingly delicious. You can put it on top of your eggs or chicken, or even eat it with veggies like raw carrots and celery!

Ingredients:

2 cans stewed tomatoes

½ white onion

1 tsp minced garlic

1 lime

1 tsp salt

1 jalapeno

½ bunch of cilantro

Directions:

1. Chop your jalapeno, onion, and cilantro finely. Juice your lime.
2. In a blender, place all ingredients into the blender. Blend on high speed until all combined.
3. Serve with your favorite vegetables, with eggs, or over chicken.

Chapter 20: Questions and Answers

While what you can eat or drink will depend a lot on your diet, the general rule of thumb is to either fast completely from food or stick to less than 500 calories throughout the fasting day. In order to stay under your limit during your fast, you need to eat and drink healthy. For drinks, try to focus on consuming a lot of plain water. You can add fruit or lemon slices to your water to help flavor it. You can also drink as much seltzer water as you would like (it is a much healthier item compared to soda!). If you want more than water, coffee and tea are also allowed. Try to keep your coffee as black as possible and only sweeten it with a splash of milk. Do not sweeten your tea. You can also drink diet soda since it is calorie free (but be aware of the harmful effects of artificial sweeteners). For food, stick to lean protein and lots of fruits and vegetables. On your fasting days you want to avoid high calorie items, even if they are healthy, because you will often still end up hungry and your calorie count could go over. Raw veggies like carrots and celery are easy snacks that are healthy and will fill you up with little calories. Also leafy greens like kale and romaine lettuce can make a great salad with some grilled chicken breast on top. Skip the dressing and use some balsamic vinegar to toss your greens in. You want to focus on eating healthy and whole foods so that you can continue to stay satisfied while keeping under your calorie limit.

Will I get hungry?

You can bet on that!

Imagine that your body has been used to eating meals at frequent intervals at every 4 hours for the past 30 years and then comes a sudden switch to a totally different eating windows at every 24 hours. It can surely send your body confusing havoc signals. But worry not! This is only a temporary phase when your body is trying to adjust. There are many ways to smoothen this transitional change and minimize the hunger effects. Read on to the next FAQ for more tips.

Do understand the difference between physical and emotional hunger as well. Only when you are able to distinguish between two, you can then know how to manage and react in the correct manner. Here are some characteristics of the two type of hungers.

Physical Hunger:

- Comes on gradually and can be postponed
- Can be satisfied with any type of food without specific cravings
- Once full, stops eating automatically
- Causes satisfaction

Emotional Hunger:

- Comes on suddenly and feels urgent
- Causes specific food cravings
- Eat more than normal and feel uncomfortably full
- Causes guilty feeling

While intermittent fasting can have an adjustment period in the beginning where you will feel hungry, this often subsides as time goes on. Many forms of intermittent fasting have been shown to lower your insulin, leptin, and ghrelin levels so that you are not as hungry throughout the day and you become satisfied with food much quicker. However, this change is not immediate. When you start fasting and are not used to it, you will most likely feel the hunger. Try to remember that there is a difference between hunger and food cravings. You are often feeling hungry only because you have trained your brain to want food at certain times of the day. If you space out your snacks and keep to healthy and low-calorie options, you will feel less hungry. There will be fewer instances where you feel hungry as time goes on.

What should I do when I get hungry?

If you are fasting and you start to feel hungry, try the tips below. Remember that this hunger is temporary. You should not be feeling hungry all the time!

Drink Water

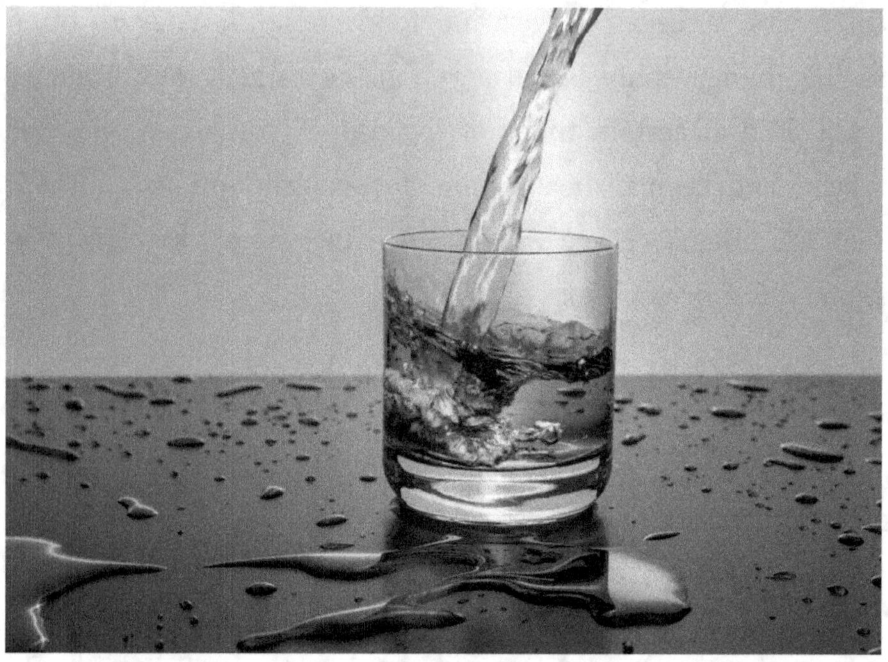

This might sound obvious and brought up repeatedly. Your brain will signal your body when you are thirsty to eat food. This is because you get a lot of your water from food you eat as well. Drinking a glass of water may take this hunger away.

Drink Sparkling Water

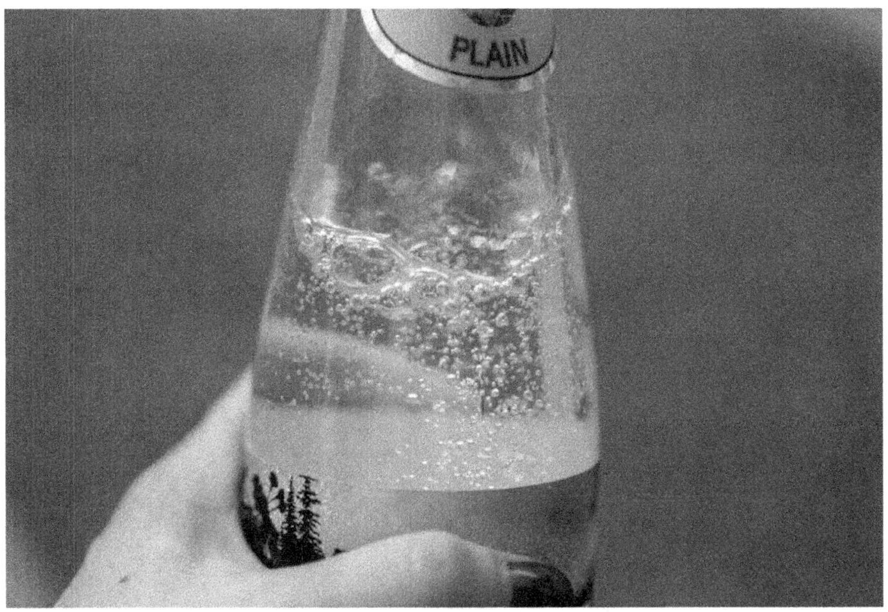

Similar to drinking plain water, drinking sparkling water can give a full feeling to your stomach. Sparkling water can make you feel fuller and gives you the mental relief with the naturally flavored ones. Just make sure that you choose the zero calorie sparkling water.

Drink Black Coffee

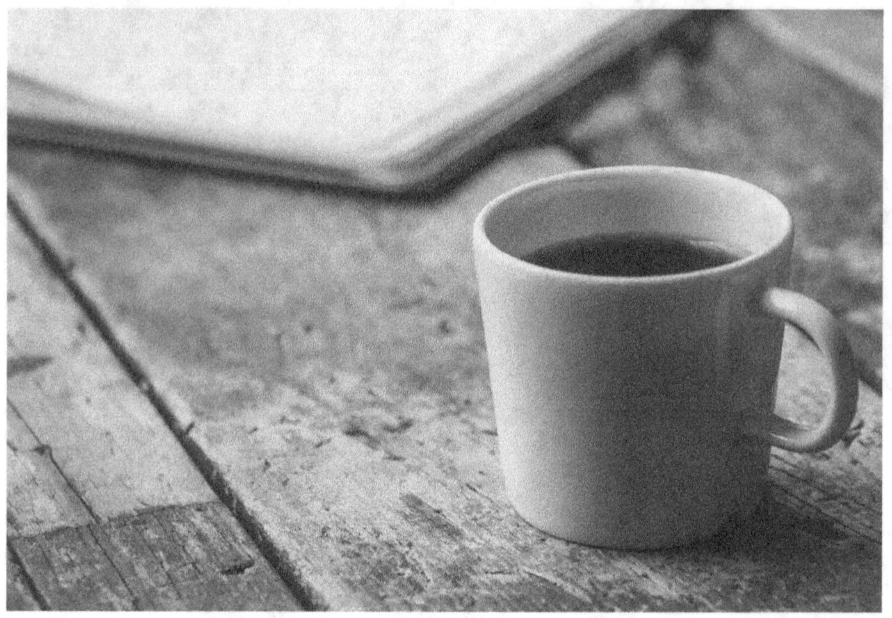

If you are a frequent coffee drinker with milk and sugar, drinking black coffee may need some getting used to. Black coffee is commonly recommended as the caffeine helps with appetite suppression. You may start your day with 2 cups of black coffee after waking up if you are on LeanGains 16/8 fasting method.

Drink Hot Bone Broth

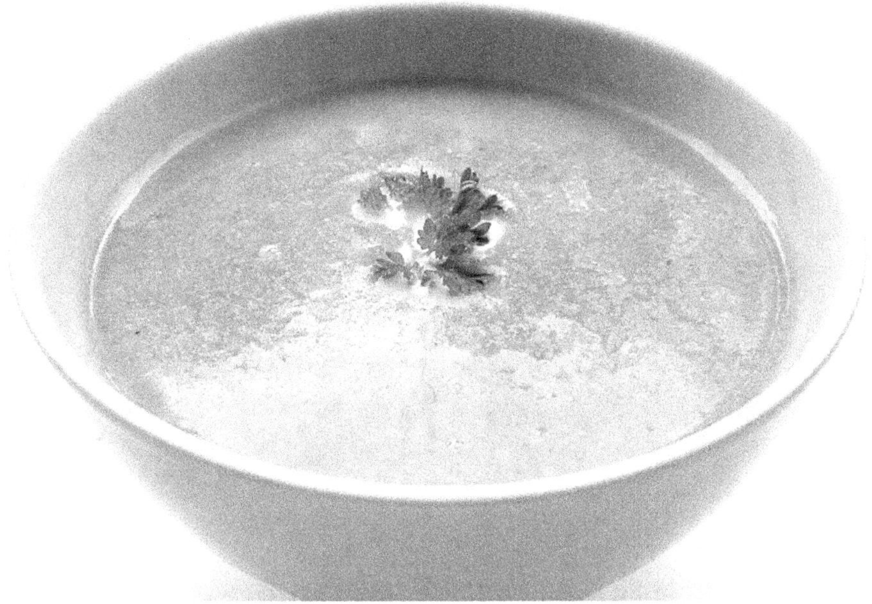

Depending on the fasting method, bone broth may be allowed. One cup of bone broth typically contains about 30 to 50 calories. Hence, it is quite minimal and brings little impact to the overall calorie intake as compared to other food. However, bone broth is rather costly and it "technically" break the fast due to its calorie. Hence, it is wise to have this as your last few resorts when you are absolutely struggling.

Chew Sugar-Free Gum

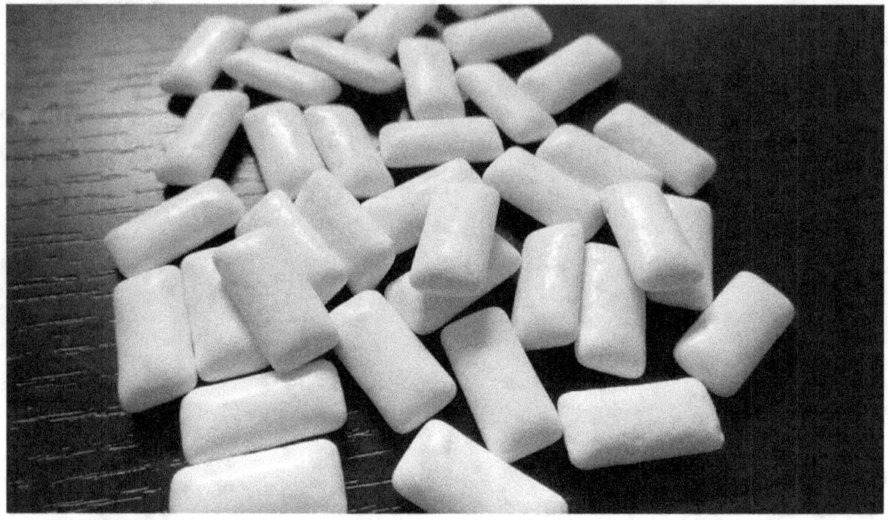

Yes, we might have been pretty desperate to resort to this cheap trick after trying all drinks allowable by intermittent fasting. By chewing gum, the slow release of the flavor and the chewing action, may keep you satisfied for some time.

Focus on a Task

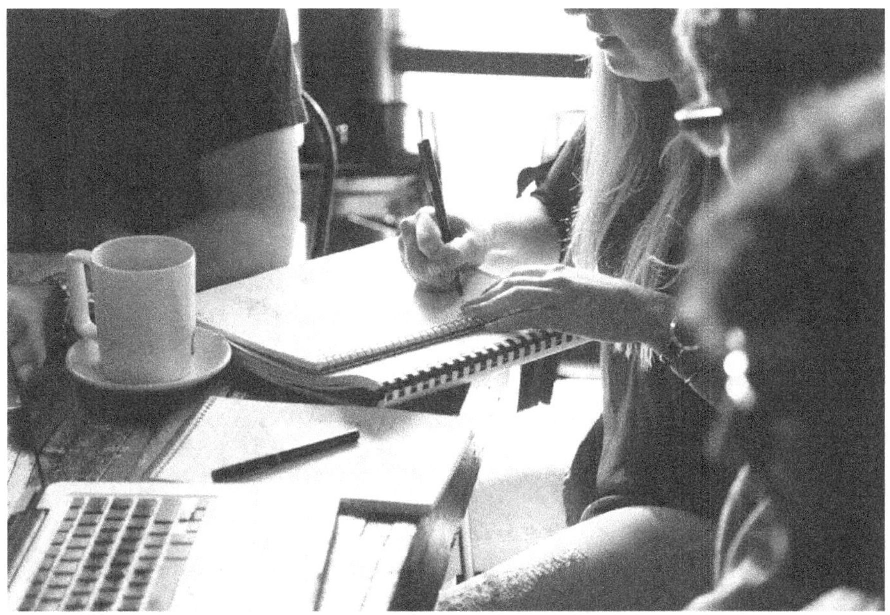

Rough periods of fasting can be good time to get serious work completed. With your mind engaged on something that excites you or requires your full focus, it may be easier to get through the hunger fog.

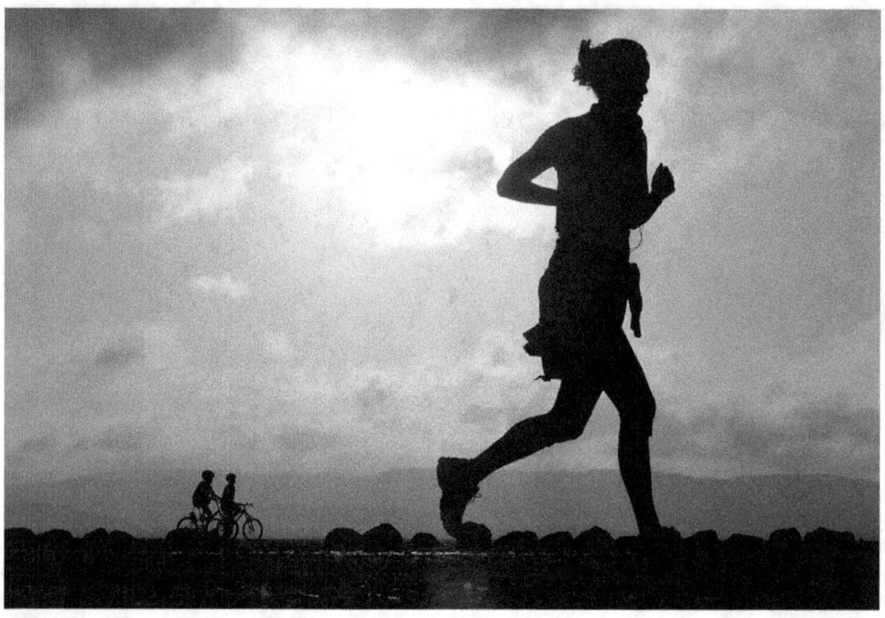

Most people may think that one should hibernate and conserve energy during fasting. However, it is actually the opposite. Our bodies tend to be more efficient at reaching out for the energy stores when we are active as we move around. Working out with weights works on the same logic as well.

Meditation

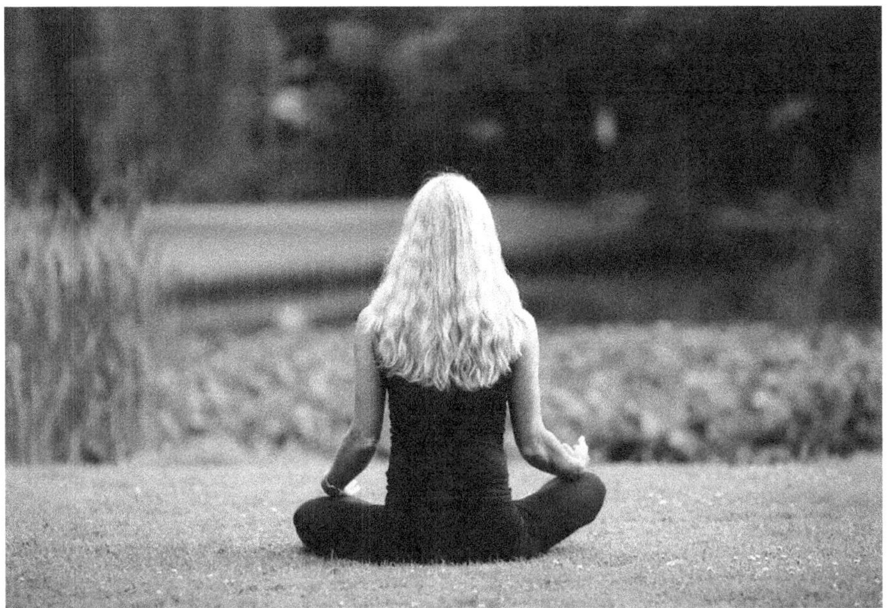

By practicing mindfulness, it may help to clear our mind and detach any urge from eating. Though this may not work for everyone, its surely worth a shot given the numerous proven benefits that come with meditation.

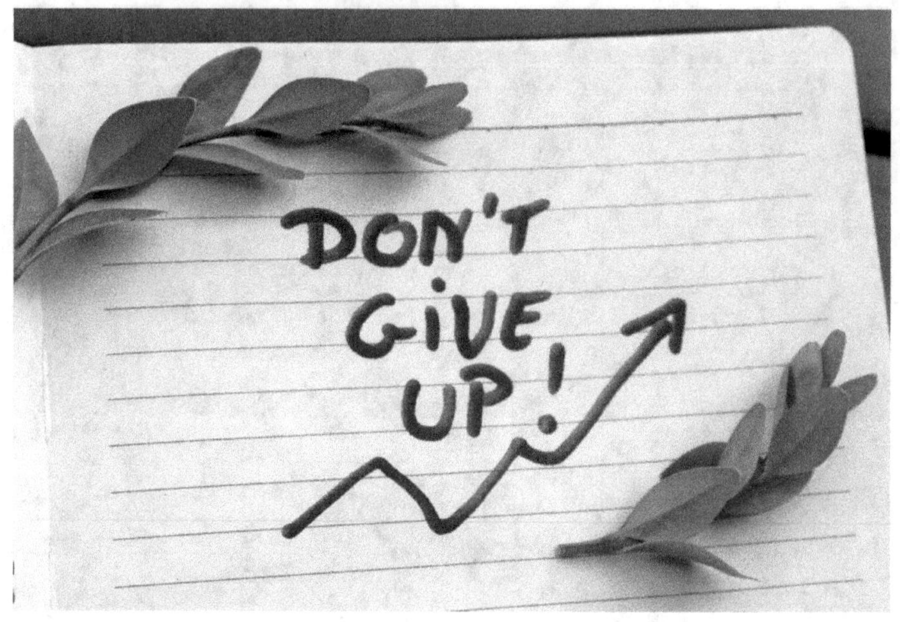

When in doubt, recall why you started the intermittent fasting journey. You definitely started fasted for a good reason. You probably didn't stop eating just for the sake of not eating. Hence, it is strongly encouraged that you pen down your personal reasons for starting on fasting and what you aim to achieve after 6 months. Write down as elaborately as possible and have this note prominently displayed so that you can be reminded every day.

The bigger your "Why", the more willing you will grind through the difficult times.

Some people believe that if you do not have food in your body while working out that you are going to faint or pass out. While you may feel light-headed while working out in your fasted state, this is temporary. It usually only happens when you are a beginner at intermittent fasting. Once your body gets used to fasting, you will no longer feel like this. It is not dangerous to work out in a fasted state. In fact, many of the benefits of intermittent fasting come from working out in a fasted state. Take it slow the first few times you work out without food. Soon enough your body will adjust and you will not notice a difference. If you feel over-exhausted, reduce your work out intensity and slow down. Ensure that you are sufficiently hydrated as well.

Where do I get my energy from for my workouts?

When you work out with food in your stomach, your body burns carbohydrates. While this is not bad, you are only burning the calories you had just eaten. When you work out in a fasted state, your energy comes from your stored adipose tissue. This adipose tissue holds your stored fat. Hence, you start to burn through your fat stores as you work out in fasted state. Fat has been shown to give you longer lasting energy than the carbohydrates your body usually burns. And the added benefit is that you are burning more fat than you would if you work out after eating. If you are looking to lose weight or burn excess fat you may have, you should see better results by working out in a fasted state.

This is the question that many people have on intermittent fasting. The short answer is no, you will not lose muscle from fasting. When you follow a traditional diet of restricting calories, you will lose weight. However, when you lose weight from traditional dieting you lose fat and muscle. Research has shown that this does not happen on intermittent fasting diets. It has actually been shown to help you gain muscle if you work out in addition to fasting. This is why intermittent fasting is often popular among gym goers. You do not only burn your body fat, you are also going to convert that fat into muscle by working out and fasting.

When your body goes into starvation mode, your metabolism shuts down and you hold onto your fat stores for future use. When you fast, your body does not go into starvation mode because it is not remaining starved long enough. When you restrict your calories every day, your body thinks it is not getting enough calories and not consistently enough. When you only restrict your calories one or two days a week, you are not stopping your metabolism long enough for your body to go into starvation mode. This is a good thing! When you fast, you are putting your cells under stress. Your cells then adapt better to future stress and they work harder and stronger. Also, your metabolism speed does not drop. This is a common problem on a traditional dieting regimen. You lose weight from restricting calories but you are not restricting calories often enough to stop your metabolism and slow it down. There is one study that found alternate day fasting for 22 days did not lead to any drop in metabolic rate, instead, the participants shown 4% fat mass reduction.

Hence, the takeaway is that metabolism scientifically increases during fast of up to 48 hours.

No one likes being left out. It is one of the main complaints about trying to fast. One of the easiest ways to remedy this problem is to fast on days that are not busy and that does not potentially coincide with social events. This may typically mean it is probably not best to fast on the weekends. Now obviously it is not realistic to fast on a day with no social events for forever. But, choosing days that usually do not have social events is much easier for your fasting routine. Also, certain intermittent fasting diets will not have this problem as much as others. If you often go to dinner with friends, the warrior diet or LeanGains will not interfere with that. But, if you go to breakfast or brunch often then the warrior diet and LeanGains diet would interfere. If you cannot avoid fasting for the social event, you have two options. You can either fast through it or decide to break your fast early or skip it. If it is a one-time event, it is okay to occasionally skip the fasting. This diet should not become so strict that you are obsessed with the tiny details. But, if you do not want to skip this diet there are some things you can do. First, stay away from the food! Talk and mingle with your friends. Focus on the company you are surrounding yourself with and forget about the food! Food is not your life. If you are going to socialize, do it. Socialize! If the food is at the beginning of the event, show up later. If it is at the end of the event, leave the event early. It is easy to avoid the food at social events. You can also talk to your family and friends about your fasting. If you tell them all the benefits and show them this book, they too might want to start an intermittent fasting routine!

My family/friends/colleagues think that intermittent fasting is crazy and unhealthy. How can I convince them?

First things first, share the benefits with them using your personal experience. People who think fasting is unhealthy are often unfamiliar with how fasting works and how your body responds to it. Second, show them this book! Invite them to read this book for quick understanding of the science behind intermittent fasting. It can be discouraging to sustain a diet or routine that others are constantly trying to bring down. Interestingly, most of the people who try to talk down on a diet often not know much about it. Explain the benefits you have experienced by fasting. By sharing your personal experience, it allows others to familiarize themselves with the diet and understand why you do it. This may just make them want to find out more and commit to intermittent fasting themselves! And if not, at least you can get them off your case like that.

An inverse yet effective approach is to ignore the funny looks and criticism from others. Why? Because results speak louder than words. Let your exuding confidence, glowing skin, overflowing positive energy, lean body and joy spread the influence on them instead. They will eventually realize and can't help but to ask you for your secret remedy. Now, that's when you can share your learnings proudly about intermittent fasting.

Chapter 21: Tips!

Ready to jump right into intermittent fasting? We have some tips that will make the whole process a lot easier for you.

First of all, do not get set on one type of intermittent fasting just from reading. You will definitely want to try a few of these methods out to truly determine the method that work best for you. We are all different and unique. While one method may work great for one person, it may be horrible for another. Listen to your body and choose the method that makes you feel the best.

Also, try to make a meal plan. When you know what you are going to eat for your fasting and non-fasting days, things become a lot easier. So many people fail at intermittent fasting because they are at a loss of what to eat on their fasting days. Having a plan ensures your day goes smoothly. You do not want to be staring at a vending machine at work wondering which snack will do the least damage to your calorie count.

Another tip is that you are going to save money! When you fast, you do not have to eat or prepare as much food. Less food equals less money spent! It is truly a win-win situation. It is wise to spend the savings the money saved on healthier food choice.

You will want to drink a lot. Water in your stomach helps your hunger and helps to trick you into thinking that you are fuller than you really are! An empty stomach is a hungry stomach. Fill that belly up with fluids!

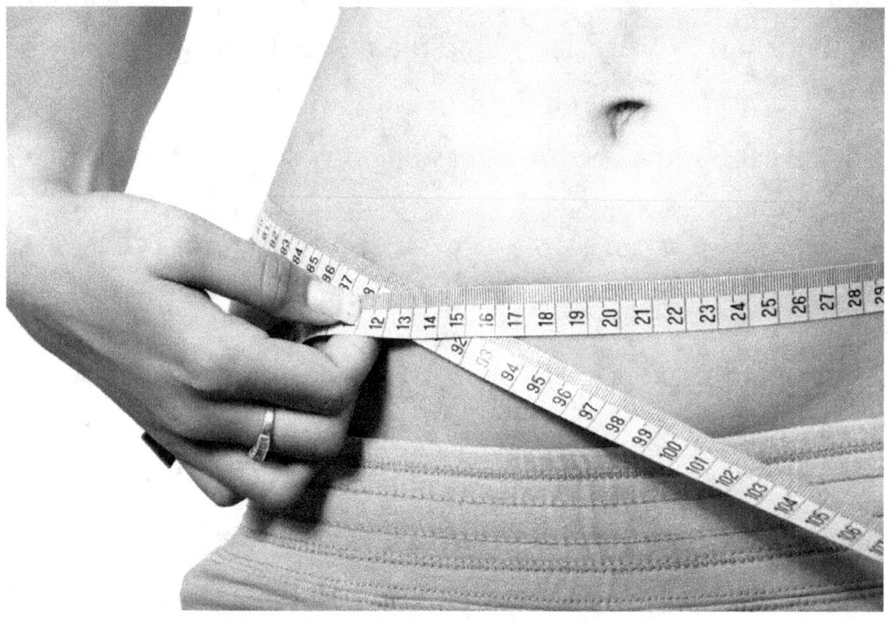

Finally, you have to try intermittent fasting for at least eight weeks. The first few weeks will be hard! Expect them to be so. Go into it knowing that your body is making a big adjustment. You are going to feel that adjustment being made. Make sure you are sticking to your fast and give it eight weeks. If you hate it, fine! But you cannot make a true opinion on it until you have done it for two months.

Conclusion

Intermittent fasting is a great way to get you healthy. It can help you to lose weight, burn away fat, and lower your insulin levels and cholesterol! It is easier to follow than your traditional calorie restrictive diets and anyone can benefit from it.

Intermittent fasting is all about meal timing. Most of these methods do not have a ton of guidelines about what to eat and whether or not you should workout. While just following the intermittent fasting protocol can lead to a healthier you, eating healthy with the right portion size and working out will allow you to have the best results possible. No matter what intermittent fasting method you choose to follow, you are on your way to a leaner you!

Once a while, if you have to break away from the routine due to other priorities, it's perfectly fine. There's no need to fret or stress over one unsuccessful fasting window. It wouldn't affect your body that much for that one occurrence of non-compliant eating window. Find the joy and fun in the intermittent fasting process so that you can enjoy it and integrate as part of your lifestyle. One unhealthy meal doesn't make you unhealthy. Conversely, one healthy meal or practice doesn't turn you healthy suddenly too. Always remember **it's the consistency that matters not the intensity.** Consistency is undeniably the key towards your intermittent fasting success!

www.ingramcontent.com/pod-product-compliance
Lightning Source LLC
Chambersburg PA
CBHW061352250726
48657CB00004B/1460